Dermatological Manifestations of the Lower Extremity

Editor

TRACEY C. VLAHOVIC

CLINICS IN PODIATRIC MEDICINE AND SURGERY

www.podiatric.theclinics.com

Consulting Editor
THOMAS ZGONIS

July 2016 • Volume 33 • Number 3

ELSEVIER

1600 John F. Kennedy Boulevard • Suite 1800 • Philadelphia, Pennsylvania, 19103-2899

http://www.theclinics.com

CLINICS IN PODIATRIC MEDICINE AND SURGERY Volume 33, Number 3
July 2016 ISSN 0891-8422, ISBN-13: 978-0-323-44854-3

Editor: Jennifer Flynn-Briggs
Developmental Editor: Alison Swety

Clinics in Podiatric Medicine and Surgery (ISSN 0891-8422) is published quarterly by Elsevier Inc., 360 Park Avenue South, New York, NY 10010-1710. Months of issue are January, April, July, and October. Business and Editorial Offices: 1600 John F. Kennedy Blvd., Ste. 1800, Philadelphia, PA 19103-2899. Customer Service Office: 3251 Riverport Lane, Maryland Heights, MO 63043. Periodicals postage paid at New York, NY and additional mailing offices. Subscription prices are $285.00 per year for US individuals, $498.00 per year for US institutions, $100.00 per year for US students and residents, $370.00 per year for Canadian individuals, $602.00 for Canadian institutions, $435.00 for international individuals, $602.00 per year for international institutions and $220.00 per year for Canadian and foreign students/residents. To receive student/resident rate, orders must be accompanied by name of affiliated institution, date of term, and the signature of program/residency coordinator on institution letterhead. Orders will be billed at individual rate until proof of status is received. Foreign air speed delivery is included in all Clinics subscription prices. All prices are subject to change without notice. POSTMASTER: Send address changes to Clinics in Podiatric Medicine and Surgery, Elsevier Health Sciences Division, Subscription Customer Service, 3251 Riverport Lane, Maryland Heights, MO 63043. **Customer Service: 1-800-654-2452 (US). From outside of the US, call 314-447-8871. Fax: 314-447-8029. E-mail: JournalsCustomerService-usa@elsevier.com (for print support); JournalsOnlineSupport-usa@elsevier.com (for online support).**

Reprints. For copies of 100 or more of articles in this publication, please contact the Commercial Reprints Department, Elsevier Inc., 360 Park Avenue South, New York, NY 10010-1710. Tel.: 212-633-3874; Fax: 212-633-3820; E-mail: reprints@elsevier.com.

Clinics in Podiatric Medicine and Surgery is covered in MEDLINE/PubMed (Index Medicus) and EMBASE/Excerpta Medica.

CLINICS IN PODIATRIC MEDICINE AND SURGERY

CONSULTING EDITOR
THOMAS ZGONIS, DPM, FACFAS

Contributors

CONSULTING EDITOR

THOMAS ZGONIS, DPM, FACFAS
Professor and Director, Externship and Reconstructive Foot and Ankle Fellowship Programs, Division of Podiatric Medicine and Surgery, Department of Orthopaedics, University of Texas Health Science Center San Antonio, San Antonio, Texas

EDITOR

TRACEY C. VLAHOVIC, DPM, FFPM RCPS (Glasg)
Clinical Associate Professor, Department of Podiatric Medicine, J. Stanley and Pearl Landau Faculty Fellow, Temple University School of Podiatric Medicine, Philadelphia, Pennsylvania

AUTHORS

CHRIS G. ADIGUN, MD
Board Certified Dermatologist and Nail Specialist, Pinehurst Skin Surgery Center, Pinehurst, North Carolina

CHRIS BOWER, MB ChB, FRCP
Consultant Dermatologist, Department of Dermatology, Royal Devon and Exeter NHS Foundation Trust, Exeter, United Kingdom

IVAN BRISTOW, PhD, FFPM RCPS (Glasg)
Senior Lecturer, Faculty of Health Sciences, University of Southampton, Southampton, United Kingdom

NATHANIEL J. JELLINEK, MD
Fellowship Director, Micrographic Surgery and Dermatologic Oncology, Dermatology Professionals, Inc, East Greenwich, Rhode Island; Assistant Clinical Professor, Department of Dermatology, Warren Alpert Medical School, Brown University, Providence, Rhode Island; Adjunct Assistant Clinical Professor, Division of Dermatology, University of Massachusetts Medical School, Worcester, Massachusetts

M. TARIQ KHAN, PhD, BSc PodMed, BSc (Hons), MChS, FCPM, FFPM RCPS (Glasg)
Consultant Podiatrist and Director, Marigold Clinic, The Royal London Hospital for Integrated Medicine, University College London Hospital NHS Foundation Trust; Hon. Research Fellow, Department of Dermatology, Barts Health Trust; Consultant Podiatrist, EB Department, Great Ormond Street Hospital for Sick Children, London, United Kingdom; Hon. Senior Lecturer, St. George Medical School, University of New South Wales, New South Wales, Australia; Clinical Adjunct Professor, Department of Podiatric Medicine, Temple University School of Podiatric Medicine, Philadelphia, Pennsylvania

LEON H. KIRCIK, MD
Clinical Associate Professor of Dermatology, Indiana University School of Medicine; Mount Sinai Medical Center, New York, New York; Physicians Skin Care, PLLC, Louisville, Kentucky

STEPHEN M. SCHLEICHER, MD
Director, DermDOX Center for Dermatology, Hazleton, Pennsylvania; Clinical Director, DermDOX Podiatry-Dermatology Fellowship, St. Luke's Health Systems, Bethlehem, Pennsylvania; Associate Professor of Medicine, The Commonwealth Medical College, Scranton, Pennsylvania; Adjunct Assistant Professor of Dermatology, University of Pennsylvania Medical College, Philadelphia, Pennsylvania

NICOLE F. VÉLEZ, MD
Westmoreland Dermatology Associates, Monroeville, Pennsylvania

JOSEPH VELLA, DPM, AACFAS
Private Practice, Impression Foot and Ankle, Gilbert, Arizona

TRACEY C. VLAHOVIC, DPM, FFPM RCPS (Glasg)
Clinical Associate Professor, Department of Podiatric Medicine, J. Stanley and Pearl Landau Faculty Fellow, Temple University School of Podiatric Medicine, Philadelphia, Pennsylvania

Contents

> Onychomycosis is the most common nail disease seen in podiatric practice. Effective long-term management remains problematic. We need to treat onychomycosis effectively to prevent its progression into a severe, debilitating, and painful condition, and to manage recurrence. With new agents now available and greater discussion on management strategies, this article reviews the appropriate evaluation of the disease, treatment options, and optimal patient outcomes.

> Nail surgery is a fundamental component of podiatric surgery. Nail disorders are common and may cause significant morbidity and occasionally mortality. Diagnosis of inflammatory and infectious conditions, and of benign or malignant tumors, often requires a biopsy of the nail unit. Excisional surgery may also be curative for certain tumors. This article reviews key elements of nail anatomy, surgical preparation, local anesthesia, and methods to achieve and maintain a bloodless field. A familiarity with these concepts should allow clinicians to develop a surgical plan and approach when patients present with a nail disorder requiring biopsy or surgical treatment.

> Viral warts or verruca pedis (plantar warts) are common skin conditions seen in both children and adults. Human papilloma virus (HPV), a DNA virus, is responsible for plantar verrucae. It needs an epidermal abrasion and a transiently impaired immune system to inoculate a keratinocyte. These entities are a therapeutic conundrum for many practitioners. This article discusses HPV infiltration and its subtypes involved in plantar warts; the evaluation of patients with plantar warts; and subsequent treatment options, such as laser, *Candida albicans* immunotherapy, topical therapy such as phytotherapy, and surgical excision.

Melanoma is a rare form of skin cancer that is responsible for most skin cancer deaths globally. Tumors arising on the foot continue to be a particular challenge. Patients present later and lesions are frequently misdiagnosed, leading to more advanced disease with an overall poorer prognosis then melanoma elsewhere. In order to improve early recognition, this article reviews the clinical features of the disease along with published algorithms. Emerging assessment techniques such as dermoscopy are also discussed as tools to improve clinical decision making. Contemporary drug therapies in the treatment of advanced disease are also discussed.

The skin of the lower extremity can be a helpful diagnostic tool for systemic disease. Diabetes, renal disease, genetic disorders, and even cancer can have cutaneous manifestations in the legs and feet; moreover, proper diagnosis can facilitate earlier treatment of these diseases and not only clear up the skin symptoms but also bring about resolution of the systemic disease causing them. Although not comprehensive, this article discusses many of these disorders presenting with integumentary manifestations in the lower extremities. Where appropriate, it also enumerates the treatments involved, both systemic and localized.

Plantar hyperhidrosis, excessive sweating on the soles of feet, can have a significant impact on patients' quality of life and emotional well-being. Hyperhidrosis is divided into primary and secondary categories, depending on the cause of the sweating, with plantar hyperhidrosis typically being primary and idiopathic. There is an overall increased risk of cutaneous infection in the presence of hyperhidrosis, including fungal, bacterial, and viral infections. This article discusses a range of treatment options including topical aluminum chloride, iontophoresis, injectable botulinum toxin A, glycopyrrolate, oxybutynin, laser, and endoscopic lumbar sympathectomy. Lifestyle changes regarding hygiene, shoe gear, insoles, and socks are also discussed.

CLINICS IN PODIATRIC MEDICINE AND SURGERY

RELATED INTEREST

Primary Care: Clinics in Office Practice, December 2015 (Vol. 42, Issue 4)
Primary Care Dermatology
George G.A. Pujalte, *Editor*
Available at: http://www.primarycare.theclinics.com/

THE CLINICS ARE AVAILABLE ONLINE!
Access your subscription at:
www.theclinics.com

Foreword

Lower Extremity Skin Manifestations

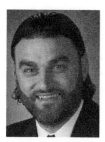

Thomas Zgonis, DPM, FACFAS
Consulting Editor

This issue of *Clinics in Podiatric Medicine and Surgery* is dedicated to pathological skin conditions of the lower extremity. Various topics from plantar verrucae, psoriasis, fungal infections, hyperhidrosis, and melanoma lesions are well covered in a comprehensive manner by our expert Guest Editor, Dr Vlahovic, and invited authors. Equal attention is emphasized on common adverse drug reactions of the lower extremities as well as lower extremity cutaneous manifestations based on systemic diseases. Last, surgical procedures on the skin and nail disorders are also well included in this issue.

Dermatologic conditions of the lower extremity are very common in our practices, and I am grateful to our authors for completing this multidisciplinary issue from all related specialties. In addition, I would like to thank all of our readers, editorial board members, and authors for their continuous support and outstanding submissions.

Thomas Zgonis, DPM, FACFAS
Division of Podiatric Medicine and Surgery
Department of Orthopaedics
University of Texas Health Science Center
San Antonio
7703 Floyd Curl Drive-MSC 7776
San Antonio, TX 78229, USA

E-mail address:
zgonis@uthscsa.edu

Clin Podiatr Med Surg 33 (2016) xi
http://dx.doi.org/10.1016/j.cpm.2016.04.002
0891-8422/16/$ – see front matter © 2016 Published by Elsevier Inc.

podiatric.theclinics.com

Preface

Lower Extremity Skin Manifestations: A Multidisciplinary Effort

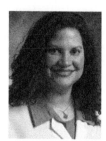

Tracey C. Vlahovic, DPM, FFPM RCPS (Glasg)
Editor

I am pleased to bring you a joint effort between podiatric physicians and dermatologists to update you on lower-extremity dermatologic conditions. I gathered the best in the field to show the partnership, camaraderie, and interplay that exist between podiatric medicine and dermatology. Podiatric dermatology is extremely relevant to our daily practice, yet often feared and misunderstood due to the similarities in presentation and overwhelming differential diagnoses. As I am passionate about all things podiatric dermatology-wise, I chose topics that I felt the practitioner would benefit from in everyday practice. In this issue, you can explore everything from choosing the best topical medication for a fungal infection from a vehicle perspective by Dr Kircik to manifestations of systemic disease by Dr Vella. Drs Jellinek and Vélez offer a fascinating primer on nail surgery, and Drs Bristow and Bower provide insight on lower extremity melanoma. My former attending physician and textbook coauthor, Dr Schleicher, discusses various treatments for psoriasis ranging from topical to systemic. Drug reactions, which are often overlooked and misdiagnosed on the lower extremity, are discussed in depth by Dr Adigun. I had the opportunity to work with Dr Khan on writing everything about plantar verruca. I round out this podiatric dermatologic smorgasbord with topics on therapies for onychomycosis, plantar hyperhidrosis, and pediatric dermatologic concerns.

I am extremely grateful to all who contributed. You are leaders in your field, and it has been an honor to work with you. I am hoping you, the reader, gain insight and

Clin Podiatr Med Surg 33 (2016) xiii–xiv
http://dx.doi.org/10.1016/j.cpm.2016.04.001
0891-8422/16/$ – see front matter © 2016 Published by Elsevier Inc.

appreciate their efforts as several of these topics are being presented in the podiatric literature for the first time.

Tracey C. Vlahovic, DPM, FFPM RCPS (Glasg)
Department of Podiatric Medicine
Temple University School of Podiatric Medicine
148 North 8th Street
Philadelphia, PA 19107, USA

E-mail address:
traceyv@temple.edu

Onychomycosis

Evaluation, Treatment Options, Managing Recurrence, and Patient Outcomes

Tracey C. Vlahovic, DPM, FFPM RCPS (Glasg)

KEYWORDS

- Onychomycosis • Efinaconazole • Tavaborole • Laser • Toenail
- Trichophyton rubrum • Mycosis • Tinea pedis

KEY POINTS

- Onychomycosis is a common disease that requires effective management to prevent progression to a severe and debilitating condition.
- Confirming the diagnosis of onychomycosis is paramount especially before starting a systemic medication.
- Onychomycosis can be managed with either topical or systemic agents, and new topical agents afford better options to tailor appropriate therapy for our patients.
- Combination therapy (topical and systemic) may be an important consideration in more difficult to treat patients. Prophylaxis with topical agents may help prevent disease recurrence.
- Treatment of coexisting tinea pedis is critical and a number of strategies may be used to minimize the long-term consequences of the disease.

INTRODUCTION

Onychomycosis is a common superficial fungal infection of the nails leading to discoloration, nail plate thickening, and onycholysis. Mycotic nail disease is the most common nail pathology worldwide, reaching all cultures and ethnicities. Onychomycosis is increasing, accounting for up to 90% of toenail and at least 50% of fingernail infections.[1] The most common etiology in the United States is owing to dermatophytes, typically *Trichophyton rubrum* and *Trichophyton mentagrophytes*.[2] In Europe, *T rubrum* is the chief agent followed by *T mentagrophytes* and *T interdigitale*.[3,4] Nondermatophyte molds and yeasts also play a role with varying frequency.

Disclosures: Advisor, speaker and investigator for Valeant and Pharmaderm.
The authors acknowledge Brian Bulley, MSc, of Inergy Limited for medical writing support. Valeant Pharmaceuticals North America LLC funded Inergy's activities pertaining to this article.
Department of Podiatric Medicine, Temple University School of Podiatric Medicine, 148 North 8th Street, Philadelphia, PA 19107, USA
E-mail address: traceyv@temple.edu

Clin Podiatr Med Surg 33 (2016) 305–318
http://dx.doi.org/10.1016/j.cpm.2016.02.001
0891-8422/16/$ – see front matter © 2016 Elsevier Inc. All rights reserved.

Because the initial diagnosis is predicated on the nail's appearance, the diagnostic gold standard is direct microscopy (potassium hydroxide [KOH]) and fungal culture. However, visual nail plate changes are used to classify onychomycosis,[5] including distal subungual (also known as distal lateral subungual onychomycosis [DLSO], the most common form), proximal subungual, superficial white, and total dystrophic.[6]

Onychomycosis occurs in 10% of the general population, 20% of individuals 60 years and older, and 50% of individuals over 70 years.[6] Peripheral vascular disease, immunologic disorders, and diabetes mellitus correlate with the increased prevalence in older adults. The risk of onychomycosis is 1.9 to 2.8 times greater in persons with diabetes mellitus, and in patients with HIV infection prevalence rates range from 15% to 40%.[6] Other predisposing factors include older age, sex (male > female), genetic predisposition, tinea pedis (interdigital or moccasin types), peripheral arterial disease, smoking, nail trauma, inappropriate nail hygiene, and family background of onychomycosis and hyperhidrosis.[6]

Adult patients constitute the bulk of those seeking treatment, but there are increasing numbers of pediatric cases, possibly owing to increasing childhood obesity and pediatric diabetes. With prevalence ranging from 0% to 2.6% worldwide, pediatric onychomycosis is relatively rare compared with adults, but still one of the most common nail disorders in children.[7] DLSO is the most common type seen in children, followed by proximal subungual and white superficial. The most common pathogen is *T rubrum*.

In the last several years, novel treatments and considerations regarding the diagnosis and management of onychomycosis have arisen. This review discussed emerging conservative and surgical methods to treat the disease.

PATIENT EVALUATION

To evaluate a patient presenting with nail dystrophy, the practitioner should begin by completing a thorough history and physical evaluation. With treatment options ranging from systemic to surgical, knowledge of medical history, current medications, and family history will aid in the differential diagnosis and formulating the treatment plan. Key questions include: how long have you had the nail changes, is it painful, has it affected your quality of life? Daily shoe gear choices, work and athletic activities, and the home and work environments will all assist treatment plan selection. Level of immunosuppression, vascular status, and the ability to take oral or apply topical medication should be taken into account. Discussion and examination of any other skin rashes or conditions should be completed, because psoriasis and eczema can mimic mycotic nails.

Visual assessment is imperative. Since the Zaias classification was proposed in 1972, modifications have been proposed and published to reflect the wide array of dermatophytes, nondermatophyte molds, and yeasts as well as the complications of various patterns occurring in the same nail or other inflammatory diseases copresenting with mycosis.[8] Nail plate changes include DLSO where the invasion begins at the hyponychium and disturbs the distal nail bed; proximal subungual, where invasion begins proximally; superficial white, where the upper surface of the nail plate is first attacked[8]; total dystrophic, which describes total nail plate involvement and surrounding periungual tissue; and endoynx, which describes distal nail plate attack resulting in a deeper penetration of hyphae.

In addition, the physician should determine how many toenails are involved on 1 or both feet, percent involvement of the nail, any biomechanically aggravating factors that could contribute to nail dystrophy (adductovarus fifth digit, hammertoe, or hallux abductovarus), and the presence of tinea pedis interdigitally or plantarly.

Approximately 50% of nail disease is caused by onychomycosis[9]; the remainder conditions that mimic onychomycosis, having similar signs and symptoms, include psoriasis, lichen planus, reactive arthritis, allergic/irritant contact dermatitis, and eczema. Other differential diagnoses include alopecia, nail changes secondary to biomechanical issues, melanoma (and other skin cancers), traumatic onycholysis, 20-nail dystrophy, and pachyonychia.[10–12]

Because not all presenting nail disease is mycotic, it is important to confirm with laboratory diagnosis if the treatment plan includes oral antifungal therapy, if there is concomitant skin disease difficult to distinguish in the nails, and if the patient has been on antifungal therapy previously and disease has recurred. Laboratory diagnostic methods include direct microscopy (KOH test), nail plate biopsy for periodic acid Schiff stain, and fungal culture. Generally, KOH and fungal culture are done together; KOH shows the presence of hyphae, and culture the species present. Unfortunately, fungal cultivation is a slow process ($\leq$4 weeks) and may generate false-negative results in 40% of the cases that are microscopically positive.[13] As an alternative periodic acid Schiff stain involves sending nail plate (commonly referred to as, but not a true, biopsy) for staining to determine presence of dermatophytes. Periodic acid Schiff staining provides quicker results and is more sensitive, whereas culture is more specific (regarding species).[14–16]

Standard mycological tests, KOH, and fungal culture may yield false-negative or false-positive results, and require time to verify the pathogens.[17] Accurate diagnoses are often delayed owing to lack of both specific and rapid methods of pathogen identification. When the mycological analyses are negative and the clinical picture is highly suggestive of onychomycosis, polymerase chain reaction (PCR) testing may be an option.[18] Antifungal drug efficacy and dosages may differ for different causative pathogens, and it has been hypothesized that mixed and nondermatophyte onychomycosis may be cause for high rate of treatment failures.[19] A rapidly sensitive method for detection and identification will better guide an appropriate treatment strategy. PCR detects a specific DNA sequence; moreover, fungi species-specific PCR diagnostic methods are available,[20,21] deepening our understanding and treatment of onychomycosis.[22] Because DNA is extremely resistant and can persist even in the absence of viable hyphae, DNA amplification techniques such as PCR may represent a useful addition to standard procedure.[23] Time will tell how truly beneficial PCR will be both in the physician office and in clinical trials.

PHARMACOLOGIC TREATMENT OPTIONS: FOCUS ON TOPICAL THERAPY

Onychomycosis can be managed with topical or systemic agents. The current standard of care is an oral antifungal agent (either terbinafine or itraconazole) because they are more effective than topical agents, owing to issues of penetrance into the nail apparatus with topical agents. Drug interactions and the risk of hepatic injury may limit their desirability, especially in the elderly where the disease is most prevalent.

Guidelines suggest monotherapy with topical antifungals is limited to:

- Superficial white, except in transverse or striate infections,
- DLSO, except in the presence of longitudinal streaks, when less than 80% of the nail plate is affected with lack of involvement of the lunula, or
- When systemic antifungals are contraindicated.[24]

Developing effective topical treatments for onychomycosis has been complicated by low permeation rates through the nail plate to the site of infection.[25–28] The nail may be more permeable to agents formulated in an aqueous vehicle.[29] Unlike ciclo-pirox and amorolfine nail lacquers, new topical agents, efinaconazole and tavaborole, are now available as solutions.

Studied in separate trials with similar, but not identical inclusion criteria, reported complete cure rates of tavaborole were 6.5% to 9.1%.[30] Efinaconazole results were 15.2% to 17.8%.[31] Mycologic cure rates were 53.4% to 55.2% for efinaconazole, whereas the mycologic cure for tavaborole was 31.1% to 35.9% (**Table 1**). Although much emphasis has been placed on the need for active ingredient to pass through the nail plate, recent data suggest that efinaconazole may reach the infection site after transungual and subungual application[32,33]; subungual delivery data with tavaborole is pending.

Lacquer-based topical therapies are applied primarily to the exterior nail plate, with the drug reaching the infection site mostly through nail permeation.[34–36] Efinacona-zole is applied to the clean, dry nail plate surface, lateral and proximal nail folds, hyponychium, and undersurface of the nail plate.[37] Application to the hyponychium and ventral aspect of the nail plate may be important in patients wishing to continue to use nail polish.[32] Although nail polish does not seem to influence efinaconazole penetration into the nail, it can become tacky with repeated application.[38] Up to 4 layers of nail polish does not seem to inhibit penetration of tavaborole either.[39] In neither case has the impact of nail polish on efficacy been assessed, nor is it contraindicated.

Because toenail growth progresses from proximal to distal, newly formed nail plate replaces diseased nail, a process that can take 12 to 18 months.[39] Clinical trial data suggest that tavaborole and efinaconazole must be applied daily to the toenails for at least 48 weeks. Some patients may require treatment for considerably longer because of slow toenail growth, disease severity, or for other reasons. It is not known whether longer treatment regimens with tavaborole or efinaconazole would produce better efficacy results; however, higher cure rates after longer follow-up periods have been reported with other agents.[40–42]

It is important that patients recognize that cure may not translate to a completely clear nail.[43] Poor adherence with any long-term chronic therapy is well documented.[44] A number of post hoc analyses with efinaconazole have been carried out to better identify prognostic factors for treatment success. Gender[45] and disease severity[46] were significant influencers of complete cure over the duration of the studies; female patients and those with milder disease may see results much quicker in clinical prac-tice, whereas male patients and those with moderately severe disease may require a longer treatment course, or combination therapy with oral antifungals. Although male patients are more difficult to treat, reasons are unclear. They tend to seek help for more advanced disease and suffer more nail trauma, and their toenails tend to be thicker. The reduced rate of growth and thickness of the nail may be factors in more severe disease, although it may be that these patients just require longer treat-ment courses.

Tinea pedis is an important causative factor for onychomycosis, and better results are seen when any coexisting tinea pedis is also treated.[47] In addition, managing tinea pedis is critical to minimizing disease recurrence.

Onychomycosis remains a common, progressive, and difficult disease to manage successfully. Early diagnosis and treatment are important irrespective of risk factors or comorbidities.[48] A multidirectional approach to drug delivery may broaden the utility of topical therapies, such as efinaconazole in the treatment and greater clinical expe-rience will help to guide management practice.

Table 1
Efficacy results from recent clinical trials with efinaconazole and tavaborole in mild to moderate onychomycosis

Cure	Efinaconazole Clinical Studies[31]				Tavaborole Clinical Studies[30]			
	Efinaconazole (n = 656)	Vehicle (n = 214)	Efinaconazole (n = 580)	Vehicle (n = 201)	Tavaborole (n = 399)	Vehicle (n = 194)	Tavaborole (n = 396)	Vehicle (n = 205)
Complete (%)	17.8	3.3	15.2	5.5	6.5	0.5	9.1	1.5
Mycologic (%)	55.2	16.8	53.4	16.9	31.1	7.2	35.9	12.2

Complete cure and mycologic cure rates after 48 weeks' daily therapy, 4-week follow-up data (*P*<.001 for all active data vs respective vehicle data).

NONPHARMACOLOGIC TREATMENTS

Debridement, the mechanical reduction of toenail length and thickness using nail nipper or rotating burr, may provide a valuable adjunct for patients experiencing pain upon ambulation and in shoe gear.[49] Although debridement alone improves quality of life and nail thickness, it does not result in mycological cure.[50] Topical ciclopirox and debridement improved patient's quality of life and resulted in mycologic cure.[50] However, debridement added to oral antifungal therapy may offer a only a small benefit.[51,52] Debridement can provide pain relief and improved patient satisfaction, affording an opportunity to encourage adherence. It may offer benefits through reduced fungal load, and enhanced penetration of topical drugs into the nail unit. For patients who opt against pharmacologic treatment, debridement will allow more comfort in shoe gear and reduce potential pressure on the nail bed, especially if diabetic neuropathy is present.

Nail avulsion, the separation of the nail plate from the nail bed, can be achieved nonsurgically with daily application of topical 40% urea for 1 to 2 weeks.[53] Generally, this is followed by application of a topical antifungal once the toenail has been removed, repeating as necessary. It is more common in Europe.[53] Nail avulsion can be useful in patients who have a needle/procedure phobia, who have peripheral vascular disease or another comorbidity precluding pharmacologic intervention, or have a single nail infected. However, removal of the nail itself will not result in clearance of the infection, even when followed by topical antifungal therapy.

Management of onychomycosis is a long-term challenge for some patients owing to the rate of recurrence and reinfection. Many do not want to add another oral medication to their regime, or use a daily topical product for a year. Laser therapy is a nonsurgical, nonpharmacologically based option. Approved devices include Nd:YAG 1064 nm lasers and a diode at 870/930 nm.[54] The US Food and Drug Administration approved laser treatment of certain wavelengths to "temporarily improve the appearance of the nail," making no claims regarding mycological cure owing to device approval being based on substantial equivalence to already existing devices on the market.[54] The mechanism of action is unknown, but proposed to be bulk heating of the nail unit selectively destroying fungal elements.[54] In the onychomycosis laser studies, the definition of "cure" and number of treatments are extremely variable, and the fluence (energy applied per surface area) differs from device to device. Consistency within studies on mycological diagnosis varies, and strictness of a pharmaceutical clinical trial lacking. It is difficult to extrapolate settings used on the nail, the length of treatment, and outcomes owing to the differences in just the Nd:YAG laser class. Most likely patients who opt to receive laser as monotherapy will need several treatments over a 12- to 16-month period owing to the lack of recurrence data and possibility for reinfection.[54,55] It has potential as an adjunct to both oral and topical antifungals, but further research is needed to show efficacy.

COMBINATION THERAPY

New topical antifungals and device-based therapies have expanded therapeutic options in onychomycosis. Combination therapy with multiple drug classes and routes of administration may improve overall efficacy especially in patients proven difficult to treat successfully with more traditional methods.

The rationale for the combination of topical and oral therapy in the treatment of onychomycosis is that systemic antifungals reach the infection via the nail bed, and topical agents are absorbed through the nail surface.[56] In addition, some topical agents may reach the site of infection via the hyponychium. Ideally, combined antifungals should be synergistic in their mode of action and specific activity against the types of fungal infection seen in onychomycosis.

Combination therapy can be used sequentially or in parallel. In patients likely to fail therapy (ie, those with diabetes or having yellow spikes in the nail), parallel treatment is invaluable. Sequential treatment (ie, treating initially with an oral agent and following up with topical treatment) may be helpful in patients who show a poor response to treatment.[57]

Combination therapy with oral and lacquer-based topical antifungals has been shown to lead to a marked improvement of mycological and clinical outcomes associated with onychomycosis,[35,43,58,59] and may be more cost effective than using a systemic agent alone.[43] Currently, there are no data with the newer solution-based topical agents (eg, efinaconazole and tavaborole) used in combination with an oral agent to treat onychomycosis and data are eagerly awaited given the apparent superior efficacy as monotherapy. Data on the combined use of an oral agent and laser therapy also suggest a more rapid and effective clinical outcome in patients with onychomycosis.[60]

SURGICAL TREATMENT OPTIONS

For a singularly painful or thickened nail, some patients may opt for total nail removal. Surgery involves application of local anesthesia to the digit followed by removal of the nail plate in toto. Simple total avulsion of the nail itself is not curative for a mycotic nail, because the procedure does not address the basis of infection. Combining nail avulsion and topical antifungals has been described as the preferred treatment plan. Total nail avulsion with the use of a topical azole cream applied twice-daily to the exposed nail bed resulted in a high dropout rate. All patients with total dystrophic onychomycosis failed, and only 56% of patients (15/27) were cured with this approach,[61] suggesting that the procedure should not be generally suggested for the treatment of onychomycosis.

Nail avulsion has been suggested to obtain a better specimen for fungal culture, but should only be used in situations where both systemic and topical antifungal therapies have failed.[53] Contraindications include patients with peripheral vascular disease, autoimmune disorders, collagen vascular disease, diabetes, hemostasis disorders, and acute infection/inflammation of the periungual tissue.[62] Possible keratinization of the nail bed as the nail plate is growing is also a concern.

MANAGEMENT OF RECURRENCE

Despite the number of available treatment options, not all onychomycosis patients are cured, or will remain cured. Recurrence (either as a result of relapse or reinfection) is not uncommon, seen in 10% to 53% of patients[63]; rates increase with increasing post-treatment period.

Several factors may play a role although it is not known which are the most important:

- Family history;
- Age;
- Occupation;
- Lifestyle;
- Environmental conditions;
- Underlying nail physiology (ie, presence of a very thick nail, extensive involvement of the entire nail unit, lateral nail disease and yellow spikes);

- Physical trauma, especially in the elderly;
- Concomitant disease (eg, peripheral vascular disease and diabetes);
- Presence of tinea pedis; and
- Immunosuppressed patients.

Only coexisting diabetes mellitus has been shown to have a significant negative impact on recurrence rates ($P = .026$).[60] Although recurrence rates were higher with greater nail involvement (>50%; $P = .01$) and age (>60 years; $P = .18$), these were not significant.[64]

Few studies have followed the clinical course of patients beyond 12 months after systemic or topical therapy.[65,66] With systemic therapy, recurrence has been shown to be more common with itraconazole than terbinafine, although in both cases the rates increase with posttreatment interval.[67,68] Mean time to recurrence after successful treatment was 36 months in a 7-year prospective study of 73 successfully treated onychomycosis patients.[66] Other factors, including presence of predisposing factors, use of nail lacquer as a prophylactic treatment, and isolated dermatophyte strain were not related significantly to relapse.[66] The long-term benefits of terbinafine are probably related to its fungicidal action, compared with the fungistatic action of itraconazole.[69]

There are no good data on recurrence rates with topical therapy, where follow-up after cessation of treatment in clinical trials was limited to 4 weeks. Data from the clinical trials on efinaconazole and tavaborole show complete cures rates continuing to increase posttreatment, suggesting recurrence may not a problem in the immediate term. A study of 207 patients successfully cured and followed for 12 months after completion of therapy included 6 patients treated with amorolfine nail lacquer. Recurrence rates (33.3%) were similar to those seen with terbinafine (38.5%) and itraconazole (34.3%).[64]

Data on the prevention of recurrence with topical therapy is limited. A small open-label study (n = 52) with amorolfine prophylaxis in patients previously cured with terbinafine or terbinafine and amorolfine showed statistical significant results compared with untreated controls ($P = .047$). These data suggest a modest benefit that does not seem to be sustained. Relapse rates at month 12 were 8.3% and 31.8% respectively; however, by month 36 differences were not significant, and had occurred in 29.2% of the patients treated prophylactically with twice-weekly amorolfine.[70] A 2-year study in 48 patients found that biweekly use of miconazole powder 2% to prevent recurrence showed no difference between active and placebo.[70] A subsequent case report was able to demonstrate sustained remission from onychomycosis with once-weekly miconazole cream applied to the affected toe and toe clefts.[71]

The optimal dosing regimen or duration of prophylaxis with topical agents is unknown, although data from other long-term recurrence studies with systemic treatments suggest 2 to 3 years.[72] Amorolfine prophylaxis was dosed twice weekly, and it is not known whether more frequent dosing would have resulted in greater protection from recurrence.[66] Amorolfine can be detected in the nail for about 2 weeks, and normal dosing to treat onychomycosis is to apply to the nail plate once or twice a week.[73] High concentrations of efinaconazole have been shown to remain in the nail plate for at least 2 weeks after cessation of therapy,[74] suggesting the potential for twice weekly prophylaxis. The lack of benefit beyond 12 months may be a function of poor adherence, or infrequent dosing.

Prophylaxis in diabetic patients with onychomycosis would seem to be very important, given the high relapse potential and risk of complications. In addition to treating immediate family members to help spread of disease, encouraging patients prone to tinea pedis to self-treat is critical.

EVALUATING PATIENT OUTCOMES AND LONG-TERM MANAGEMENT

There have been a number of discussions of onychomycosis cure in the literature; yet there remains no agreement on definition of treatment success.

The clinical trial definition of complete cure is probably too stringent.[75,76] A consensus conference proposed 2 alternative criteria: 100% absence of clinical signs of onychomycosis (mycology not required), or negative mycological laboratory results with 1 or more of the following clinical signs: distal subungual hyperkeratosis or onycholysis leaving less than 10% of nail plate affected, or nail plate thickening that does not improve with treatment because of comorbid condition.[2] More recently, it has been suggested that absence of clinical signs after an adequate washout period, coupled with negative culture, with our without negative microscopy, should be considered as a cure.[76]

These definitions raise a number of important considerations. In some patients, complete cure may not be a realistic option, and yet both physician and patient may be still happy with the outcome. In addition, a longer treatment duration (12–18 months) may produce a better clinical outcome; however, adherence may become a significant issue.[77] Longer washout periods of 3 to 6 months, while allowing for the removal of both residual drug and nonviable fungal cells to afford a more accurate interpretation of mycological outcome, increase the risk of recurrence.[77]

Evaluating clinical outcomes should be done with reference to baseline severity, and patients are encouraged to take pictures of their toenails at regular intervals. Because it is also common for other toenails to be affected, and occasionally both feet, it has been suggested that efficacy should be based on clinical improvement in all involved onychomycotic toenails.[78]

Patient outcomes in onychomycosis after appropriate treatment are generally good. There are some patients who will never have a completely clear nail, or nails. Others do not respond to topical or systemic antifungal therapy; reasons may be multifactorial and unclear. In some cases, combination therapy or repeated courses of antifungals may be required.

Given that it may be 12 to 18 months before the nails grow out fully, and the significant treatment commitment, long-term recommendations to maintain clear nails are important. In controlled clinical trial environments recurrence rates are very high and increase with posttreatment interval. In clinical practice the number of onychomycosis patients suffering recurrence is likely to be higher, with suboptimal treatment. However, there are a number of steps patients can take to minimize risk. Prophylactic use of antifungal agents should be encouraged on a regular basis for patients suffering persistent infection. Twice weekly applications may be effective, although it is not certain whether prophylaxis beyond 1 year is cost effective or desirable without other preventative measures. Treating other family members with the disease, and treating any tinea pedis is likely to minimize recurrence significantly.

In addition, footwear and sock decontamination remain an important consideration because these items can act as a fungal reservoir. It has been shown that at least 10% of patients with tinea pedis and onychomycosis are at risk of reinfection by contact with their socks.[79] Footwear can be decontaminated with antifungals, ultraviolet light, or potentially ozone.[80–83] Patients should also try to avoid activities known to risk spread of disease such as swimming and washing clothes (especially socks) in cold water.[84]

Successful treatment of onychomycosis can be a challenge and long-term recommendations are critical in such a chronic, recurring condition. A number of strategies, both therapeutic and practical can be used successfully.

SUMMARY

In the past 2 years, onychomycosis has become a hot topic again in both podiatric medicine and dermatology owing to the introduction of 2 new topical antifungals (efinaconazole and tavaborole). As these are novel agents in treating mycotic nails, it also allows one to go back and revisit the other options already available: systemic, nonsurgical, and surgical. With the vast amount of therapeutic possibilities out there (that also have an array of cure rates and complications), it is important for the clinician to choose the best option for the patient's situation and nail disease. Of most importance, confirming the diagnosis of onychomycosis is paramount, especially before starting a systemic medication. Choosing other modalities to treat the nail, whether as monotherapy or as a combination regime, should be tailored to each patient. Overall, the clinician has more options than ever to manage fungal nail disease and ultimately improve quality of life for these patients.

REFERENCES

1. Ghannoum MA, Hajjeh RA, Scher R, et al. A large-scale North American study of fungal isolates from nails: the frequency of onychomycosis, fungal distribution, and antifungal susceptibility patterns. J Am Acad Dermatol 2000;43:641–8.

2. Thomas J, Jacobson GA, Narkowicz CK, et al. Toenail onychomycosis: an important global disease burden. J Clin Pharm Ther 2010;35(5):497–519.

3. Borman AM, Campbell CK, Fraser M, et al. Analysis of the dermatophyte species isolated in the British Isles between 1980 and 2005 and review of worldwide dermatophyte trends over the last three decades. Med Mycol 2007;45:131–41.

4. Saunte DM, Svejgaard EL, Haedersdal M, et al. Laboratory-based survey of dermatophyte infections in Denmark over a 10-year period. Acta Derm Venereol 2008;88:614–6.

5. Zaias N. Onychomycosis. Dermatol Clin 1985;3(3):445–60.

6. Westerberg DP, Yoyack MJ. Onychomycosis: current trends in diagnosis and treatment. Am Fam Physician 2013;88(11):762–70.

7. Gupta AK, Skinner AR, Baran R. Onychomycosis in children: an overview. J Drugs Dermatol 2003;2:31–4.

8. Hay RJ, Baran R. Onychomycosis: a proposed revision of the clinical classification. J Am Acad Dermatol 2011;65:1219–27.

9. Faergemann J, Baran R. Epidemiology, clinical presentation and diagnosis of onychomycosis. Br J Dermatol 2003;149(Suppl 65):1–4.

10. Murphy F, Jiaravuthisan MM, Sasseville D, et al. Psoriasis of the nail: anatomy, pathology, clinical presentation, and review of the literature on therapy. J Am Acad Dermatol 2007;57(1):1–27.

11. Rich P, Elewski B, Scher RK, et al. Diagnosis, clinical implications, and complications of onychomycosis. Semin Cutan Med Surg 2013;32(2 Suppl 1):S5–8.

12. Moll JM. Seronegative arthropathies in the foot. Baillieres Clin Rheumatol 1987; 1(2):289–314.

13. Fletcher CL, Hay RJ, Smeeton NC. Onychomycosis: the development of a clinical diagnostic aid for toenail disease. Part I. Establishing discriminating historical and clinical features. Br J Dermatol 2004;150:701–5.

14. Weinberg JM, Koestenblatt EK, Tutrone WD, et al. Comparison of diagnostic methods in the evaluation of onychomycosis. J Am Acad Dermatol 2003;49(2): 193–7.

15. Reisberger EM, Abels C, Landthaler M, et al. Histopathological diagnosis of onychomycosis by periodic acid-Schiff-stained nail clippings. Br J Dermatol 2003; 148(4):749–54.
16. Borkowski P, Williams M, Holewinski J, et al. Onychomycosis: an analysis of 50 cases and a comparison of diagnostic techniques. J Am Podiatr Med Assoc 2001;91(7):351–5.
17. Elewski BE. Diagnostic techniques for confirming onychomycosis. J Am Acad Dermatol 1996;35:56–60.
18. Arca E, Saracli MA, Akar A, et al. Polymerase chain reaction in the diagnosis of onychomycosis. Eur J Dermatol 2004;14:52–5.
19. Pierard GE, Arrese-Estrada J, Pierard-Franchimont C. Treatment of onychomycosis: traditional approaches. J Am Acad Dermatol 1993;29:S41–5.
20. Spreadbury C, Holden D, Aufaurre-Brown A, et al. Detection of aspergillus fumigatus by polymerase chain reaction. J Clin Microbiol 1993;31:615–21.
21. Miyakawa Y, Mabuchi T, Kagaya K, et al. Isolation and characterization of a species-specific DNA fragment for detection of Candida albicans by polymerase chain reaction. J Clin Microbiol 1992;30:894–900.
22. Baharaeen S, Vishniac HS. 25S ribosomal RNA homologies of basidiomycetous yeasts: taxonomic and phylogenetic implications. Can J Microbiol 1984;30:613–21.
23. Walberg M, Mørk C, Sandven P, et al. 18S rDNA polymerase chain reaction and sequencing in onychomycosis diagnostics. Acta Derm Venereol 2006;86:223–6.
24. Ameen M, Lear JT, Madan V, et al. British Association of Dermatologists' guidelines for the management of onychomycosis 2014. Br J Dermatol 2014;171:937–58.
25. Thatai P, Sapra B. Transungual delivery: deliberations and creeds. Int J Cosmet Sci 2014;36:398–411.
26. Kobayashi Y, Miyamoto M, Sugibayashi K, et al. Drug permeation through the three layers of the human nail plate. J Pharm Pharmacol 1999;51:271–8.
27. Gupta AK, Joseph WS. Ciclopirox 8% nail lacquer in the treatment of onychomycosis of the toenails in the United States. J Am Podiatr Med Assoc 2000;90:495–501.
28. Bohn M, Kraemer K. The dermatopharmacologic profile of ciclopirox 8% nail lacquer. J Am Podiatr Med Assoc 2000;90(10):491–4.
29. Hamilton JB, Terada H, Mestler GE. Studies of growth throughout the lifespan in Japanese: growth and size of nails and their relationship to age, sex, heredity, and other factors. J Gerontol 1955;10(4):401–15.
30. Elewski BE, Rich P, Wiltz H, et al. Efficacy and safety of tavaborole topical solution, 5%, a novel boron-based antifungal agent for the treatment of onychomycosis: results from two randomized phase 3 studies. J Am Acad Dermatol 2015; 73(1):62–9.
31. Elewski BE, Rich P, Pollak R, et al. Efinaconazole 10% solution in the treatment of toenail onychomycosis: two phase 3 multicenter, randomized, double-blind studies. J Am Acad Dermatol 2013;68:600–8.
32. Elewski BE, Pollak RA, Pillai R, et al. Access of efinaconazole topical solution, 10%, to the infection site by spreading through the subungual space. J Drugs Dermatol 2014;13:1394–8.
33. Gupta AK, Pillai RK. The presence of an air gap between the nail plate and nail bed in onychomycosis patients: treatment implications for topical therapy. J Drugs Dermatol 2015;14(8):859–63.

34. Singh G, Haneef NS, Uday A. Nail changes and disorders among the elderly. Indian J Dermatol Venereol Leprol 2005;71(6):386–92.

35. Baran R, Kaoukhov A. Topical antifungal drugs for the treatment of onychomycosis: an overview of current strategies for monotherapy and combination therapy. J Eur Acad Dermatol Venereol 2005;19(1):21–9.

36. Lecha M, Effendy I, Feuilhade de Chauvin M, et al. Treatment options—development of consensus guidelines. J Eur Acad Dermatol Venereol 2005;19(Suppl 1): 25–33.

37. Jublia (efinaconazole topical solution, 10%) [package insert]. Bridgewater, NJ: Valeant Pharmaceuticals LLC; 2014.

38. Zeichner JA, Stein Gold L, Korotzer A. Penetration of (^{14}C)-Efinaconazole solution does not appear to be influenced by nail polish. J Clin Aesthet Dermatol 2014; 7(9):45–8.

39. Vlahovic T, Merchant T, Chanda S, et al. In vitro nail penetration of tavaborole topical solution, 5% through nail polish on ex vivo human fingernails. J Drugs Dermatol 2015;14(7):675–8.

40. Del Rosso JQ. Advances in the treatment of superficial fungal infections: focus on onychomycosis and dry tinea pedis. J Am Osteopath Assoc 1997;97:339–46.

41. Sigurgeirsson B, Billstein S, Rantanen T, et al. L.I.ON. Study: efficacy and tolerability of continuous terbinafine compared to intermittent itraconazole in the treatment of toenail onychomycosis. Br J Dermatol 1999;141(Supp 56):5–14.

42. Baran R, Tosti A, Hartmane I, et al. An innovative water-soluble biopolymer improves efficacy of ciclopirox nail lacquer in the management of onychomycosis. J Eur Acad Dermatol Venereol 2009;23:773–81.

43. Baran R, Sigurgeirsson B, de Berker D, et al. A multicenter, randomized, controlled study of the efficacy, safety and cost-effectiveness of a combination therapy with amorolfine nail lacquer and oral terbinafine compared with oral terbinafine alone for the treatment of onychomycosis. Br J Dermatol 2007;157: 149–57.

44. Hay RJ. The future of onychomycosis therapy may involve a combination of approaches. Br J Dermatol 2001;145:3–8.

45. Rosen T. Evaluation of gender as a clinically relevant outcome variable in the treatment of onychomycosis with efinaconazole topical solution 10%. Cutis 2015;96(3):197–201.

46. Rodriguez DA. Efinaconazole topical solution, 10% for the treatment of mild and moderate toenail onychomycosis. J Clin Aesthet Dermatol 2015;8(6):24–9.

47. Markinson B, Caldwell B. Efinaconazole topical solution, 10%: efficacy in onychomycosis patients with co-existing tinea pedis. J Am Podiatr Med Assoc 2015; 105(5):407–11.

48. Rich P. Efinaconazole topical solution, 10%: the benefits of treating onychomycosis early. J Drugs Dermatol 2015;14(1):58–62.

49. Potter LP, Mathias SD, Raut M, et al. The impact of aggressive debridement used as an adjunct therapy with terbinafine on perceptions of patients undergoing treatment for toenail onychomycosis. J Dermatolog Treat 2007;18:46–52.

50. Malay DS, Yi S, Borowsky P, et al. Efficacy of debridement alone versus debridement combined with topical antifungal nail lacquer for the treatment of pedal onychomycosis: a randomized, controlled trial. J Foot Ankle Surg 2009;48:294–308.

51. Jennings MB, Pollak R, Harkless LB, et al. Treatment of toenail onychomycosis with oral terbinafine plus aggressive debridement: IRON-CLAD, a large, randomized, open-label, multicenter trial. J Am Podiatr Med Assoc 2006;96:465–73.

52. Markinson BC, Vlahovic TC, Joseph WS, et al. Diagnosis and management of onychomycosis: perspectives from a joint podiatry-dermatology roundtable. J Am Podiatr Med Assoc 2015. [Epub ahead of print].

53. Gupta AK, Paquet M, Simpson FC. Therapies for the treatment of onychomycosis. Clin Dermatol 2013;31(5):544–54.

54. Ortiz AE, Avram MM, Wanner MA. A review of lasers and light for the treatment of onychomycosis. Lasers Surg Med 2014;46:117–24.

55. Bristow IR. The effectiveness of lasers in the treatment of onychomycosis: a systematic review. J Foot Ankle Res 2014;7:34.

56. Evans E. The rationale for combination therapy. Br J Dermatol 2001;145:9–13.

57. Olafsson JH, Sigurgeirsson B, Baran R. Combination therapy for onychomycosis. Br J Dermatol 2003;149(Suppl 65):15–8.

58. Avner S, Nir N, Henri T. Combination of oral terbinafine and topical ciclopirox compared to oral terbinafine for the treatment of onychomycosis. J Dermatolog Treat 2005;16:327–30.

59. Rigopoulos D, Katoulis AC, Ioannides D. A randomized trial of amorolfine 5% solution nail lacquer in association with itraconazole pulse therapy compared with itraconazole alone in the treatment of Candida fingernail onychomycosis. Br J Dermatol 2003;149:151–6.

60. Xu Y, Miao X, Zhou B, et al. Combined oral terbinafine and long-pulsed 1,064-nm Nd: YAG laser treatment is more effective for onychomycosis than either treatment alone. Dermatol Surg 2014;40(11):1201–7.

61. Grover C, Bansal S, Nanda S, et al. Combination of surgical avulsion and topical therapy for single nail onychomycosis: a randomized controlled trial. Br J Dermatol 2007;157(2):364–8.

62. Pandhi D, Verma P. Nail avulsion: indications and methods (surgical nail avulsion). Indian J Dermatol Venereol Leprol 2012;78:299–308.

63. Scher RK, Baran R. Onychomycosis in clinical practice: factors contributing to recurrence. Br J Dermatol 2003;149(Suppl 65):5–9.

64. Ko JY, Lee HE, Jae H, et al. Cure rate, duration required for complete cure and recurrence rate of onychomycosis according to clinical factors in Korean patients. Mycoses 2011;54(5):384–8.

65. Heikkila H, Stubb S. Long-term results of patients with onychomycosis treated with itraconazole. Acta Derm Venereol 1997;77:70–1.

66. Piraccini BM, Sisti A, Tosti A. Long-term follow-up of toenail onychomycosis caused by dermatophytes after successful treatment with systemic antifungal agents. J Am Acad Dermatol 2010;62:411–4.

67. Watson AB, Marley JE, Ellis DH, et al. Long-term follow up of patients with toenail onychomycosis after treatment with terbinafine. Australas J Dermatol 1998;39:29–30.

68. Yin Z, Xu J, Luo D. A meta-analysis comparing long-term recurrences of toenail onychomycosis after successful treatment with terbinafine versus itraconazole. J Dermatolog Treat 2012;23:449–52.

69. Sigurgeirsson B, Olafsson JH, Steinsson JT, et al. Efficacy of amorolfine nail lacquer for the prophylaxis of onychomycosis over 3 years. J Eur Acad Dermatol Venereol 2010;24(8):910–5.

70. Warshaw EM, St Clair KR. Prevention of onychomycosis reinfection for patients with complete cure of all 10 toenails: results of a double-blind, placebo-controlled, pilot study of prophylactic miconazole powder 2%. J Am Acad Dermatol 2005;53(4):717–20.

71. Arroll B, Oakley A. Preventing long term relapsing tinea unguium with topical anti-fungal cream: a case report. Cases J 2009;2:70.
72. Sigurgeirsson B, Olafsson JH, Steinsson JB, et al. Long-term effectiveness of treatment with terbinafine vs itraconazole in onychomycosis: a 5-year blinded prospective follow-up study. Arch Dermatol 2002;138:353–7.
73. Tabara K, Szewczyk AE, Bienias W, et al. Amorolfine vs. ciclopirox – lacquers for the treatment of onychomycosis. Postepy Dermatol Alergol 2015;32:40–5.
74. Sakamoto M, Sugimoto N, Kawabata H, et al. Transungual delivery of efinacona-zole: its deposition in the nail of onychomycosis patients and in vivo fungicidal activity in the human nails. J Drugs Dermatol 2014;13(11):1338–92.
75. Scher RK, Tavakkol A, Sigurgeirsson B, et al. Onychomycosis: diagnosis and definition of cure. J Am Acad Dermatol 2007;56:939–44.
76. Ghannoum M, Isham N, Catalano V. A second look at efficacy criteria for onycho-mycosis: clinical and mycological cure. Br J Dermatol 2014;170:182–7.
77. Shemer A, Sakka N, Baran R, et al. Clinical comparison and complete cure rates of terbinafine efficacy in affected onychomycotic toenails. J Eur Acad Dermatol Venereol 2015;29(3):521–6.
78. Bonifaz A, Vazquez-Gonzalez D, Hernandez MA, et al. Dermatophyte isolation in the socks of patients with tinea pedis and onychomycosis. J Dermatol 2013; 40(6):504–5.
79. Feuilhade de Chauvin M. A study on the decontamination of insoles colonized by Trichophyton rubrum: effect of terbinafine spray powder 1% and terbinafine spray solution 1%. J Eur Acad Dermatol Venereol 2012;26:875–8.
80. Ghannoum MA, Isham N, Long L. Optimization of an infected shoe model for the evaluation of an ultraviolet show sanitizer device. J Am Podiatr Med Assoc 2012; 102(4):309–13.
81. Gupta AK, Brintnell WC. Sanitization of contaminated footwear from onychomyco-sis patients using ozone gas: a novel adjunct therapy for treating onychomycosis and tinea pedis? J Cutan Med Surg 2013;17(4):243–9.
82. Gupta AK, Brintnell W. Ozone gas effectively kills laboratory strains of Trichophy-ton rubrum and Trichphyton mentagrophytes using an in vitro test system. J Dermatolog Treat 2014;25(3):251–5.
83. Fisher E. How long do dermatophytes survive in the water of indoor pools? Der-matologica 1982;165:352–4.
84. Hammer TR, Mucha H, Hoefer D. Infection risk by dermatophytes during storage and after domestic laundry and their temperature-dependent inactivation. Myco-pathologia 2011;171:43–9.

Dermatologic Manifestations of the Lower Extremity
Nail Surgery

Nathaniel J. Jellinek, MD[a,b,c,]*, Nicole F. Vélez, MD[d]

KEYWORDS

• Nail surgery • Nail biopsy • Digital anesthesia • Complications

KEY POINTS

• To recognize both benign and malignant nail disorders that may benefit from surgical intervention.
• To acquire important concepts relating to nail surgery preparation, including the surgical prep, local anesthesia, and a bloodless field.
• To be familiar with several surgical approaches for obtaining an incisional or excisional biopsy of a nail disorder.
• To understand the role of en bloc excision for treatment of nail melanoma in situ.

INTRODUCTION: PATIENT EVALUATION OVERVIEW

Nail surgery is a core feature of podiatric dermatology. There are countless neoplastic and inflammatory disorders in which procedural intervention is required for either diagnostic or therapeutic purposes. A comfort level with these diagnoses, coupled with competence with digital anesthesia, surgical prep, acquiring and maintaining a bloodless field and hemostasis, as well a variety of surgical techniques allows clinicians to approach these patients with confidence and proficiency.

Usually a directed history can elicit the most important information when patients present with nail complaints. Although the most common question asked is often "How long has this been going on?" the authors have found that turning the question around and asking "When were your nails last normal?" usually elicits a more accurate

Disclosures: The authors have no conflicts of interest, funding sources, or prior presentations relevant to this article.
[a] Dermatology Professionals, Inc, 1672 South County Trail, Suite 101, East Greenwich, RI 02818, USA; [b] Department of Dermatology, Warren Alpert Medical School, Brown University, Providence, RI, USA; [c] Division of Dermatology, University of Massachusetts Medical School, Worcester, MA, USA; [d] Westmoreland Dermatology Associates, Monroeville, PA, USA
* Corresponding author. Dermatology Professionals, Inc, 1672 South County Trail, Suite 101, East Greenwich, RI 02818.
E-mail address: winenut15@yahoo.com

Clin Podiatr Med Surg 33 (2016) 319–336
http://dx.doi.org/10.1016/j.cpm.2016.02.002
0891-8422/16/$ – see front matter © 2016 Elsevier Inc. All rights reserved.

response. Routine preoperative questionnaires should enquire about the following: history of poor healing, Raynaud disease, smoking or prior infections, presence (and control, if applicable) of diabetes, vascular insufficiency and/or prior vascular surgery, ability of patient to reach the surgical site and perform wound care, history of infection, immune status/immunosuppression, presence of blood thinners, requirement for periprocedural antibiotics (in cases of infection prophylaxis or heart valve/ artificial joint replacement prophylaxis), and ability of patient to return for follow-up visit. Informed consent must be thorough, with specifics relating to nail surgery, including mention of more common long-term complications such as bleeding, infection, postoperative paresthesias,[1] cold sensitivity, possible need for further surgery, nail dystrophy, and less common/rare complications such as digital ischemia and infarction.

Preoperative examination of the nails should be performed with bright surgical lighting, with nail polish and other nail products removed, and with the patient initially in an elevated position so the clinician is not required to bend over for close examination. Dermoscopy may be used for longitudinal melanonychia (LM), erythronychia, and other pigmented lesions.[2–4] Occasionally transillumination[5] can localize subungual tumors, and traditional roentgenography or ultrasonography, computed tomography, or MRI may serve as adjuncts to the clinical examination in terms of disease characterization or localization.

PATHOLOGIC CONDITIONS REQUIRING NAIL SURGERY (BENIGN AND MALIGNANT TUMORS, INFLAMMATORY DERMATOSES, CONGENITAL DISORDERS)

The most common reason for nail surgery among podiatrists is ingrown nails. However, surgical treatment of this condition is not discussed in this article, although ample resources are available.[6] Similarly, nail debridement, although an essential and routine part of podiatric practice, is not discussed. Instead, this article focuses on issues relating to melanonychia, erythronychia, nail bed tumors, and inflammatory disorders than involve the nail.

LM, or brown-black discoloration along the vertical orientation of the nail plate, has a differential diagnosis that most importantly includes nail melanoma (**Fig. 1**). LM usually results from primary nail matrix melanocyte pathology, either from activation from their normally quiescent state (herein termed activation), benign proliferations (either single cell, lentiginous, or nested [in a nevus]), or a malignant process (**Figs. 2–4**). The differentiation between benign and malignant processes can be made based on cell morphology, or alternatively in some cases assisted simply by counting the concentration of melanocytes.[7] In adults, activation is the most common cause and may represent a normal finding, as in ethnic melanonychia (proportional to the degree of skin pigmentation) or association with a drug or other medical condition, either local (ie, chronic paronychia), cutaneous (ie, lichen planus), or systemic (ie, human immunodeficiency virus, Addison disease).

In all cases of melanonychia, the clinician's priority is to assess the likelihood of melanoma, focusing on particular nails involved (great toe has the highest risk on the feet), the number of digits involved (monodactylous being more concerning than polydactylous), and individual features of atypia.[8] Signs and symptoms that warrant biopsy include a new or changing brown or pink line, wide pigment, irregular and/or dark pigment (observed clinically or dermoscopically), monodactylous nail dystrophy, a nail mass, or symptoms of pain or bleeding. In general, excisional biopsy is preferable to incisional biopsy, and, in most instances, partial plate avulsion followed by the tangential (shave) techniques are the authors' surgical approach of choice (described later).

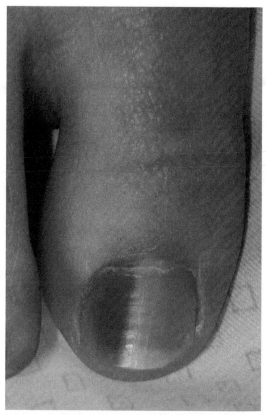

Fig. 1. LM representing nail matrix melanoma in situ. High-risk clinical features include particular digit (great toenail), width (6 mm), multiple shades of pigment. There is a suggestion of pigment of the cuticle caused by the illusory phenomenon (pseudo-Hutchinson sign).

Longitudinal erythronychia (LE) is defined as a red, vertically oriented streak in the nail and may be associated with splinter hemorrhages, distal nail splitting, distal triangular onycholysis, or distal subungual hyperkeratosis[9] (**Fig. 5**). The differential diagnosis requires an understanding of the pathogenesis, which almost always involves distal matrix disorder. The distal matrix is responsible for producing the ventral plate, so any disorder of this region, either directly involving (ie, scar, wart, squamous cell carcinoma [SCC]), indirectly involving (ie, dermal pressure from glomus tumor or subungual myxoid cyst), or alternatively inflammatory (ie, lichen planus) process can produce a nail plate thinned on the ventral surface[10] (**Box 1**). The underlying bed swells into this groove and is pinched on the sides, both of which exacerbate the normal nail bed redness and predispose to splinter hemorrhages. The distal, thinner plate is more subject to trauma, resulting in cracking, splitting, and breaking, with reactive subungual hyperkeratosis.[11] Because the differential diagnosis includes both SCC and melanoma, atypical and/or evolving lesions of LE may require biopsy.[12] Usually a partial plate avulsion and longitudinal biopsy is the surgical approach of choice (discussed later).[13]

Occasionally patients present with presumed inflammatory disorders affecting the nails, with or without more diagnostic cutaneous and/or mucosal findings. The nail

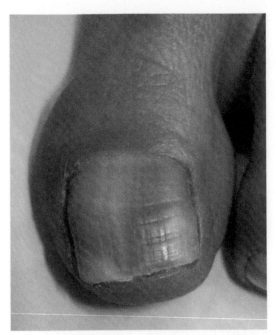

Fig. 2. Longitudinal melanonychia representing a nail matrix lentigo. The pigment is uniform, light brown-tan, without irregularity or periungual pigment.

findings may represent the only expression of disease. The most common of these diseases are psoriasis and lichen planus. Each disease may involve the matrix, the bed, both matrix and bed, and/or periungual skin (**Box 2**). Occasionally biopsy of the affected areas is indicated, and can direct appropriate therapy. For these cases,

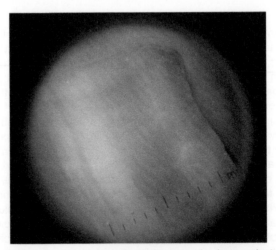

Fig. 3. Dermoscopy of clinical image from **Fig. 2** shows tan background with mostly uniform light brown lines, with darker lines of pigment proximally and suggestion of pigment dropout.

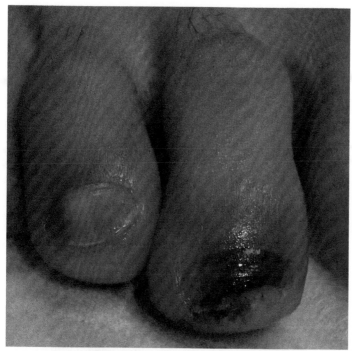

Fig. 4. Melanonychia of adjacent digits. Biopsy of the darker lesion showed melanocytic activation. There is irregular pigment and prominent periungual pigment, perhaps from activation from concurrent verruca vulgaris.

punch biopsy (of the involved area) or lateral longitudinal biopsy (including all nail subunits) is the most appropriate surgical choices (discussed later).

Congenital nail disorders are infrequent. One that is worth a brief discussion is incontinentia pigmenti (IP). An X-linked recessive disorder associated with ectodermal and musculoskeletal abnormalities, IP presents in female patients, because it is lethal to boys in utero. Cutaneous manifestations typically begin at birth with a vesiculobullous eruption that evolves into a verrucous and then macular hyperpigmentation, followed by whorled hypopigmented macular skin changes. However, occasionally the initial phase is not recognized and diagnosis is delayed. Subungual tumors may develop after puberty and can resemble SCC. Although benign, these tumors behave aggressively, can cause significant destruction to the nail bed, and a biopsy may be necessary to make an accurate diagnosis.[14–17]

SURGICAL APPROACH AND TECHNIQUES
Scrub

The foot is known to harbor a large number of resident organisms, with the corollary of higher rates of infection after orthopedic surgery on the foot and ankle than in other areas of the body. As such, the surgical scrub on the foot before nail surgery must be more thorough, ideally involve 2 different surgical prep agents, and take longer than a traditional scrub.[18–24] The authors routinely scrub with both isopropyl alcohol and chlorhexidine, prepping the area for several minutes, and use bristled brushes while applying the chlorhexidine. There is some evidence that surgical scrubs do

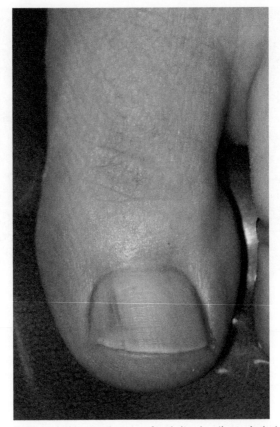

Fig. 5. LE showing light pink lines, with 1-mm focal distal nail onycholysis.

Box 1
Differential diagnosis of localized longitudinal erythronychia

Most common

- Onychopapilloma
- Scar
- Glomus tumor
- Squamous cell carcinoma/squamous cell carcinoma in situ
- Wart

Less common

- Warty dyskeratoma
- Single lesion of lichen planus
- Lichen striatus
- Subungual myxoid cyst
- Amelanotic melanoma/melanoma in situ
- Other subungual tumors (lipoma, superficial acral fibromyxoma)

Box 2
Common signs of inflammatory nail disease

Matrix disease

- Pitting
- Leukonychia
- Spotted lunula
- Grooving
- Beading

Bed disease

- Nail bed erythema
- Splinter hemorrhages
- Onycholysis
- Subungual hyperkeratosis
- Oil spots

---

not disinfect the *sub*ungual region, and that perhaps repeat scrub or simply saline wash may reduce the bacterial count after nail plate avulsion.[18] Adherence to strict sterile surgical prep is essential for all nail surgery.

Anesthesia

For most nail surgeries, either a digital (nerve) block or wing (infiltrative) block are sufficient for surgery; regional anesthesia of the foot is not required for localized surgery to the nail apparatus. The authors recently reviewed these techniques.[25] The choice of one approach rather than another is as much a matter of preference as anything else. Both deliver complete anesthesia to the nail unit and surrounding tissues. Of practical relevance, wing blocks deliver near-instantaneous anesthesia, allowing seamless transition from block to surgery, whereas digital blocks require a waiting period after injection. This wait affords an opportunity to soak the foot in warm water and chlorhexidine, a step that softens the nail plate and can facilitate nail plate manipulation.[26,27] Surgeons must beware to avoid injection of excess local anesthesia during blocks, which may result in a fluid tourniquet.

Lidocaine or ropivacaine are the two agents most commonly used. Both provide rapid anesthesia, although ropivacaine has a significantly longer duration of action and slightly longer delay to complete anesthesia. Bupivacaine is more painful during injection than either lidocaine or bupivacaine, and has a longer delay to complete anesthesia. However, injection of a long-acting anesthetic such as bupivacaine in the immediate postoperative period may give the patient long-standing postoperative pain relief and decreased need for narcotic analgesia. In this regard, ropivacaine may represent the single best agent for digital anesthesia; it has rapid onset, long duration of action, and vasoconstrictive properties that reduce bleeding.

Bloodless Field

Meticulous nail surgery cannot be performed in an excessively bloody surgical field. There are 2 widely accepted and utilized techniques to achieve temporary digital ischemia during surgery: epinephrine (mixed in dilute concentrations in local anesthesia) and/or physical pressure of the digital arteries (usually in the form of a tourniquet.) One of the authors (NJ) has commented on this in great depth.[28] Although use of epinephrine in the absence of contraindications has been shown to be safe in digital anesthesia,[29–35] is unnecessary in most cases. In nearly all nail surgeries, a vasodilatory anesthetic such as lidocaine (plain) may be used, and a temporary bloodless field produced with physical pressure on the digital arteries via manual pressure, a glove with a finger rolled back,[36] or a tourniquet.[37] As long as regimented safety procedures are followed to ensure that tourniquets are removed postoperatively, this practice ensures immediate reperfusion of the surgical field once the procedure is finished (an event that can and should be documented by the surgeon) and limits the time of digital ischemia to that of the surgical procedure itself. The authors have found that use of the glove over the foot to provide a sterile field, coupled with a glove fingertip cut off and rolled back (**Figs. 6** and **7**), works well for surgery on the great toe, and that a simple device such as the T ring is ideal for lesser toenail surgery.

Punch

Several techniques exist for sampling nail tissue and are summarized in **Table 1**. The punch biopsy is a quick and simple approach to sample the nail. It is appropriate for polydactylous inflammatory conditions, infectious disorders, LM (<3 mm wide), and for evaluation of tumors when the lesion is small. It has also proved valuable as a technique for evacuating subungual hematomas whereby the punch instrument is used to open a window in the nail plate and the hematoma is released quickly with almost

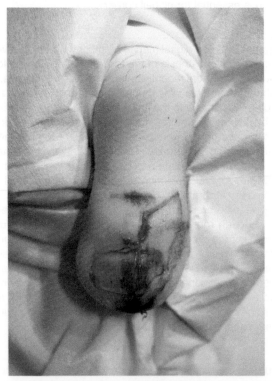

Fig. 6. Laterally located toenail LM, with a lateral longitudinal excision marked on the toe. A glove is placed over the foot with the fingertip cut and rolled back over the toe for a tourniquet.

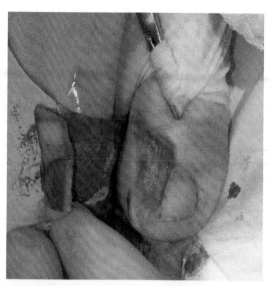

Fig. 7. Completed lateral longitudinal excision of toenail melanoma in situ (shown in **Fig. 1**). A glove is placed over the foot with the fingertip cut and rolled back over the toe for a tourniquet, with the aid of a hemostat used to grasp and turn this tourniquet mechanism for adequate hemostasis.

Table 1
Summary of nail biopsy techniques: benefits and limitations

Technique	Uses	Benefits	Limitations
Punch biopsy	• Inflammatory disorders • Infectious disorders • LM <3 mm in width • Evacuation of subungual hematoma	• Quick • No plate avulsion needed • No repair of epithelial defect required (heals by granulation) • Fast recovery	• Small sample • Risk of nail dystrophy, particularly when performed in proximal matrix
Shave biopsy (Tangential excision)	• LM or erythronychia	• Excisional biopsy of large or irregular lesions • No repair of epithelial defect required (heals by granulation) • Minimize risk of nail dystrophy	• Nail (usually partial) plate avulsion needed • Risk of nail dystrophy
Lateral longitudinal excision	• LM or erythronychia adjacent to proximal nail fold • Inflammatory conditions in which sampling of all nail subunits provides additional information	• Excisional biopsy • Sample of all nail subunits	• Greater likelihood of postoperative discomfort • Risk of postoperative cyst, spicule • Permanently narrowed nail plate • Risk of nail malalignment

immediate symptom relief.[38] Biopsies can be performed from 4 main locations: the nail folds, bed, plate, and matrix. The site is prepped in a sterile fashion and anesthesia obtained followed by establishment of a bloodless field as explained earlier.

Nail bed biopsy can be particularly informative for inflammatory disease that demonstrates bed pathology (ie, psoriasis and lichen planus) and occasionally tumors (eg, SCC, melanoma [typically the amelanotic type, when localized to the bed], and subungual epidermoid inclusions).[39] The biopsy can be performed directly through the nail plate. If nail plate avulsion is necessary for visualization/exposure of the lesion, a partial plate avulsion is preferred (discussed further later). A 3-mm punch from the nail bed is usually sufficient for diagnosis. Once the area is identified, the lesion is scored with the punch instrument. Removing the punch instrument, the surgeon examines the scored nail bed or plate and confirms the location of the biopsy. The punch is then placed in the exact location and twisted until hitting bone. Gradle scissors are inserted perpendicular to the nail bed to carefully extract the specimen (**Fig. 8**). Use of forceps should be avoided because this may crush the tissue and impair review by the

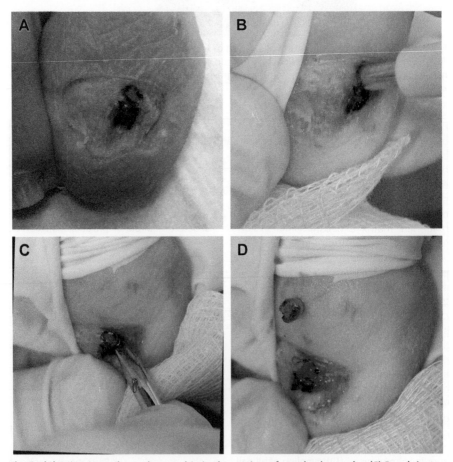

Fig. 8. (*A*) Faint, irregular melanonychia in the setting of onychodystrophy. (*B*) Punch instrument scoring over the area of pigment origin. (*C*) Gradle scissors used to extract punch specimen without the aid of forceps. (*D*) Completed punch biopsy with specimen on toe. The wound is left to heal by second intention.

pathologist.[40] A nail plate biopsy is useful in the diagnosis of proximal subungual ony-chomycosis and is performed in a similar fashion but without needing to sample the underlying epithelial tissues.

Nail matrix punch biopsy can be performed in the work-up of LM. A punch biopsy is best suited for lesions arising in the distal matrix (ie, resulting in pigment on the ventral plate) and for lesions measuring less than or equal to 3 mm. Punch biopsies of the proximal matrix and those larger than 3 mm are more likely to cause permanent split nail and are best approached with alternative methods. Dermoscopy of the lesion and the end-on distal nail plate (free edge) can help clinicians determine the origin of pigment (dorsal plate = proximal matrix, ventral plate = distal matrix). The author (NJ) previously published a more detailed discussion and algorithmic approach to evaluating LM.[28] If periungual pigment is present,[41,42] a thin sample of the cuticle and proximal or lateral nail fold should first be obtained using a 15 blade. Elevating the proximal nail fold can then expose the matrix. Tangential incisions are made on either side of the pigmented band and the proximal nail fold is undermined with an elevator, hemostat, Gradle scissors or a 15 blade. The fold is reflected back using a skin hook so that the matrix and proximal plate are exposed. The punch is then used to score and cut over the origin of the pigment, and the punch twisted until bone is reached. The specimen is carefully removed as described earlier. There is no reapproximation of the matrix defect. The proximal nail fold is returned to its original position and secured with sutures or Steri-Strips. A pressure bandage is applied and standard wound care is explained.

Shave

For LM or erythronychia that is wider than 3 mm or irregular, a 3-mm punch biopsy will only provide an incisional biopsy and risks missing the diagnosis because of sampling error. Recurrent pigment is expected. When melanoma or SCC are on the differential diagnosis, best practice includes an excisional biopsy; it provides pathologists with adequate tissue from which to make a confidant diagnosis. Although an elliptical exci-sion of the matrix is an option,[43] this can be technically challenging and more likely to cause permanent dystrophy. A shave biopsy of the nail matrix (otherwise known as a tangential matrix excision), originally described by Haneke,[44] offers an alternative approach and minimizes the risk of permanent nail dystrophy.[45]

To perform a shave biopsy of the nail matrix, the nail is first prepped in sterile fashion and local anesthesia obtained as described earlier. Again, if periungual pigment is pre-sent, a sliver biopsy of the pigmented tissue along the proximal nail fold is first per-formed and submitted as a separate specimen. Tangential incisions are then made at the junction of the proximal and lateral nail folds or at least 2 to 3 mm on either side of the pigmented lesion. The skin of the proximal nail fold is carefully undermined and the proximal nail fold is reflected proximally with a skin hook or suture. A partial proximal nail plate avulsion provides further exposure[27]: using an English anvil-action nail splitter, the clinician begins at the lateral portion of the plate at the level of the proximal one-third to one-half of the plate, and moves the nail splitter trans-versely to cut across the nail plate to the contralateral sulcus. A hemostat is used to grasp the nail plate and reflect it laterally, thus fully exposing the proximal nail bed and matrix (**Fig. 9**).

The origin of the pigmented band is identified and a 15 blade is used to score a rect-angular shape around the band with 1-mm to 2-mm margins to ensure an excisional specimen. The blade can be turned horizontally, parallel to the matrix surface, to shave the specimen using a sawing motion of the blade. A 1-mm or thinner specimen pro-vides more than adequate sampling of the matrix epithelium and dermis and does

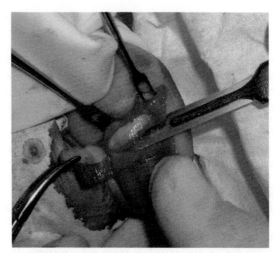

Fig. 9. Broad LM of the toe with a matrix shave biopsy. There is a partial proximal plate avulsion used to expose the proximal 50% of the nail epithelium (matrix and bed). A Penrose drain is used as a tourniquet.

not impair histopathologic review.[46] To prevent the thin shave specimen from rolling and curling, it is placed on a piece of paper in a cassette and then into a formalin jar. The specimen adheres to the paper and remains flat, thus facilitating subsequent processing.[47]

The repair is done by first trimming the laterally reflected nail plate longitudinally by 2 to 3 mm to avoid postoperative pain with tissue edema. The nail plate and proximal nail fold can then be returned to their original position. The skin of the proximal nail fold should be sutured to provide stability. The nail plate can also be sutured to the bed or the lateral nail fold. An 11 blade may be used to make holes in the nail plate to facilitate suture needle passage.

Biopsy of Longitudinal Erythronychia

As noted previously, most if not all cases of LE involve pathology of the *distal* matrix. This may be primary (direct involvement of this tissue) or secondary (as in pressure from a dermal process pushing up on the matrix); treatment of the latter involves treatment of those particular disease processes (glomus tumors, superficial acral fibromyxomas, subungual myxoid cysts). A detailed discussion of those processes is beyond the scope of this article. However, most cases of LE lack the clinical signs or patient symptoms of those processes. Most presentations represent onychopapillomas (see **Fig. 5**), although SCC in situ remains a possibility. For this more routine presentation, the biopsy is performed as follows.[13]

A trap-door or lateral curl plate avulsion is performed in routine fashion.[27] A fusiform shape is scored around the visualized lesion, extending from the mid-distal matrix to the hyponychium. This specimen is either tangential (a shave specimen) or full thickness, depending on the surgeon's preference. The authors perform these as shave specimens in most instances, removing the tissue as a specimen of less than 1 mm, similar to the matrix shave biopsy, only this includes distal matrix, bed, and hyponychium. Like the matrix biopsy, this partial-thickness wound is left to heal by second intention. With full-thickness excisional specimens, narrow defects may be left to heal by granulation, but wider specimens should be repaired, either with primary closure with undermining or with local nail flaps.[43,48] Subsequently, the nail is returned to anatomic position, sutured to the digital tip and lateral nail folds.

Lateral Longitudinal Excision

For LM or LE adjacent to the lateral nail fold or inflammatory conditions in which sampling of all nail subunits (matrix, bed, and plate) is warranted, a lateral longitudinal excision is an elegant approach.[49] However, the rate of complications, including postoperative pain, malalignment, and cyst or spicule formation, is greater with this technique than with the others previously described. For this approach, soaking the toe for 10 to 15 minutes in chlorhexidine and water, or similar antiseptic, softens the nail plate and facilitates the procedure. A scalpel blade is inserted three-quarters of the way between the cuticle and distal interphalangeal crease, 1 to 2 mm medial to the lesion, and an incision is made through the skin and soft tissue extending distally through the nail plate at the level of bone to the hyponychium on the digital tip. Starting at the same point proximally, the blade is reinserted and moved laterally around the entire horn proximally, carried through the lateral nail fold (if involved) or into the nail sulcus (if the nail fold is not involved), extending to the hyponychium and meeting the end point of the first incision (see **Figs. 6** and **7**). All incisions are to the level of bone and the ultimate result is an elliptical or curvilinear excision with margins around the lesion. Scissors and a skin hook are used to remove the specimen, with scissor tips down to avoid transection, maintain a uniform deep plane of dissection, and minimize trauma to the tissue.[47,49]

The lateral longitudinal excision should remove the entire lateral matrix horn. If small matrix remnants remain, these can produce disease recurrence, postoperative cysts, spicules, and/or pain.[50] A curette can be used to debride the lateral matrix pocket and remove any residual fragments. To repair the defect a suture is placed to realign the proximal and lateral nail fold as well as to secure the nail plate to the lateral nail fold and the distal plate to the hyponychium. Suture removal is performed at 10 to 14 days when using nonabsorbable suture material. The investigators preferentially use rapidly absorbable polyglactin 910, thus obviating suture removal.

En Bloc

En bloc excision is a technique for removing all nail tissues and can be used for excision of primary malignant nail tumors, namely SCC and melanoma in situ. It is a surgery that requires mastery of the nail unit, comfort with a bloodless field, and operating near or on the extensor tendon. Invasive melanoma in the United States is traditionally treated with digit amputation, although digit-sparing conservative approaches are being considered.[51–54] In the authors' opinion, most cases of SCC are best treated with Mohs micrographic surgery because of its high rates of cure and tissue sparing benefits.[55–60] This article therefore focuses on en bloc excision for treatment of MMIS.

During preoperative discussion and consent, it is critical that the clinician explains and documents that the en bloc procedure results in permanent nail removal and there is a risk of both positive margins and delayed recurrence requiring additional procedures, including potential amputation. The nail is then prepped as described earlier. Complete anesthesia and a bloodless field are obtained. A surgical marking pen is used to draw the planned excision margins: a transverse line is drawn at or just distal to the distal interphalangeal crease. This line is continued to the midlateral line on each side of the nail and then continues distally along the lateral nail fold, such that the two lines connect 3 to 4 mm distal to the hyponychium. The lines can be widened as needed but should not be narrowed because incomplete excision of the nail matrix increases the risk of incomplete excision, postoperative nail spicules or cysts[61] (**Fig. 10**).

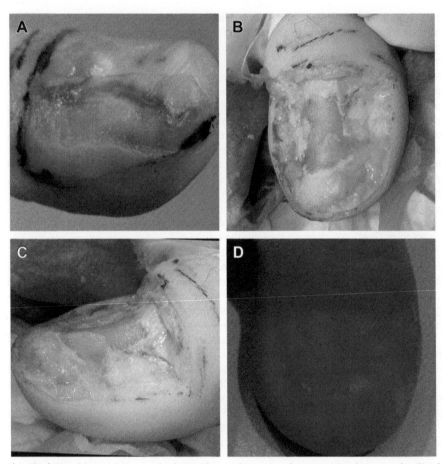

Fig. 10. (*A*) En bloc excision marked out. The markings may be as proximal as over the distal interphalangeal joint or just distal, as shown in this case. (*B, C*) En bloc excision performed at the level of the bone. (*D*) Long-term follow-up with a well-healed full-thickness skin graft.

Using a 15 blade, the lines are scored and incised. The excision plane should be at the level of the bone of the distal phalanx and over the extensor tendon and distal interphalangeal joint. Because there is no subcutaneous fat under the nail matrix and bed, dissection must be meticulous. To achieve the appropriate surgical plane, the surgeon can first approach the digit from the distal/lateral edges, using sharp dissection with a scalp blade to dissect over the ungual process of the distal phalanx, proximal to distal, so that the distal third of the bone is separated from the nail apparatus at a point where there is commonly a dorsal tuft. If the dissection starts at the tip of the digit and moves distal to proximal, the surgeon must maneuver over the ungual process and it can be difficult to keep a uniform deep plane. Instead, starting laterally/distally, the deep plane of dissection over bone is maintained. A skin hook is then used to elevate the distal nail apparatus and blunt-tipped scissors (angled tips down) are used to complete the excision.[61] The insertion of the extensor tendon is, on average, 1.2 mm proximal to the origin of the matrix and marks the end of the proximal dissection.[62] Care must be taken to complete the excision directly on the tendon (and over the joint), without causing rupture at the tendinous insertion. In practice, using scissors with fine but blunt tips (instead of a scalpel blade), bright surgical light, and loupes, and maintaining a bloodless field, all facilitate this delicate procedure and ensure clear margin excision without complication. The specimen can be oriented by inking the lateral and medial aspects of the tissue, which proves helpful in the event of a positive margin. The surgical defect is then repaired with a full-thickness skin graft (often from the upper medial arm) (see **Fig. 10**D). The defect also heals well by second intention but with a longer healing time.[63]

With experienced clinicians, the procedure works well, and is digit sparing, but close follow-up is required. Recurrences do occur and large retrospective studies with decades of follow-up are lacking. In a recent retrospective study, of 11 cases, there were 2 late local recurrences, at 7 and 11 years.[64]

COMPLICATIONS

Nail unit surgery complications are infrequent but include nail dystrophy, bleeding, postoperative pain, numbness, cyst or spicule formation, and malalignment. The most common complication of nail surgery is scarring. In a study by de Berker and colleagues[65] on outcomes of nail unit surgery in 78 patients, 22% developed postoperative scarring, such as nail splitting, ridging, or pterygium formation. Scarring usually resulted when the nail matrix had been involved in the procedure. Use of the tangential shave technique when sampling the matrix helps minimize risk of scarring.[66] Postoperative paresthesias and cold sensitivity are frequent long-term sequelae, and although not serious are irritating to many patients.

Acquired malalignment, postoperative cyst, or spicule are more common after a lateral longitudinal excision or en bloc excision. Cysts/spicules represent incomplete excision and residual remnant matrix epithelium. This complication can be avoided by ensuring complete excision of the proximal and lateral matrix horn. Postoperative bleeding is rare and can usually be controlled with pressure. Infection is also uncommon. It may present as an acute paronychia with swelling, redness, and purulence. Treatment is usually with oral antibiotics. Reflex sympathetic dystrophy has been reported in 1 patient after a nail unit biopsy.[65,67]

SUMMARY

Nail surgery is an important skill set for podiatric surgeons, with diagnostic and therapeutic implications. A variety of benign and malignant nail disorders present routinely in podiatry. By understanding the anatomy of the nail unit and options for incisional and excisional surgery, podiatric surgeons will be well prepared to approach patients who have nail disorders. As with other surgical procedures, sterile preparation, anesthesia, and a bloodless field for visualization are fundamental to obtain optimal outcomes and minimize complications.

REFERENCES

1. Walsh ML, Shipley DV, de Berker DA. Survey of patients' experiences after nail surgery. Clin Exp Dermatol 2009;34(5):e154–6.
2. Braun RP, Baran R, Saurat JH, et al. Surgical pearl: dermoscopy of the free edge of the nail to determine the level of nail plate pigmentation and the location of its probable origin in the proximal or distal nail matrix. J Am Acad Dermatol 2006; 55(3):512–3.
3. Ronger S, Touzet S, Ligeron C, et al. Dermoscopic examination of nail pigmentation. Arch Dermatol 2002;138(10):1327–33.

4. Thomas L, Dalle S. Dermoscopy provides useful information for the management of melanonychia striata. Dermatol Ther 2007;20(1):3–10.
5. Goldman L. Transillumination of fingertip as aid in examination of nail changes. Arch Dermatol 1962;85:644.
6. Haneke E. Controversies in the treatment of ingrown nails. Dermatol Res Pract 2012;2012:783924.
7. Amin B, Nehal KS, Jungbluth AA, et al. Histologic distinction between subungual lentigo and melanoma. Am J Surg Pathol 2008;32(6):835–43.
8. Braun RP, Baran R, Le Gal FA, et al. Diagnosis and management of nail pigmentations. J Am Acad Dermatol 2007;56(5):835–47.
9. De Berker D. Erythronychia. Dermatol Ther 2012;25:603–11.
10. Jellinek NJ. Longitudinal erythronychia: suggestions for evaluation and management. J Am Acad Dermatol 2011;64(1):167.e1–11.
11. de Berker DA, Perrin C, Baran R. Localized longitudinal erythronychia: diagnostic significance and physical explanation. Arch Dermatol 2004;140(10):1253–7.
12. Jellinek N, Lipner S. Longitudinal erythronychia: retrospective single center study evaluating differential diagnosis and likelihood of malignancy. Dermatol Surg 2016;42(3):310–9.
13. Collins SC, Jellinek NJ. Matrix biopsy of longitudinal melanonychia and longitudinal erythronychia: a step-by-step approach. Cosmet Dermatol 2009;22(3):19–26.
14. Mahmoud BH, Zembowicz A, Fisher E. Controversies over subungual tumors in incontinentia pigmenti. Dermatol Surg 2014;40(10):1157–9.
15. Montes CM, Maize JC, Guerry-Force ML. Incontinentia pigmenti with painful subungual tumors: a two-generation study. J Am Acad Dermatol 2004;50(Suppl 2):S45–52.
16. Malvehy J, Palou J, Mascaro JM. Painful subungual tumour in incontinentia pigmenti. Response to treatment with etretinate. Br J Dermatol 1998;138(3):554–5.
17. Simmons DA, Kegel MF, Scher RK, et al. Subungual tumors in incontinentia pigmenti. Arch Dermatol 1986;122(12):1431–4.
18. Becerro de Bengoa Vallejo R, Losa Iglesias ME, Cervera LA, et al. Efficacy of intraoperative surgical irrigation with polihexanide and nitrofurazone in reducing bacterial load after nail removal surgery. J Am Acad Dermatol 2011;64(2):328–35.
19. Bibbo C, Patel DV, Gehrmann RM, et al. Chlorhexidine provides superior skin decontamination in foot and ankle surgery: a prospective randomized study. Clin Orthop Relat Res 2005;438:204–8.
20. Ostrander RV, Botte MJ, Brage ME. Efficacy of surgical preparation solutions in foot and ankle surgery. J Bone Joint Surg Am 2005;87(5):980–5.
21. Ostrander RV, Brage ME, Botte MJ. Bacterial skin contamination after surgical preparation in foot and ankle surgery. Clin Orthop Relat Res 2003;(406):246–52.
22. Keblish DJ, Zurakowski D, Wilson MG, et al. Preoperative skin preparation of the foot and ankle: bristles and alcohol are better. J Bone Joint Surg Am 2005;87(5):986–92.
23. Brooks RA, Hollinghurst D, Ribbans WJ, et al. Bacterial recolonization during foot surgery: a prospective randomized study of toe preparation techniques. Foot Ankle Int 2001;22(4):347–50.
24. Hort KR, DeOrio JK. Residual bacterial contamination after surgical preparation of the foot or ankle with or without alcohol. Foot Ankle Int 2002;23(10):946–8.
25. Jellinek NJ, Velez NF. Nail surgery: best way to obtain effective anesthesia. Dermatol Clin 2015;33(2):265–71.
26. Jellinek NJ, Cordova KB. Frozen sections for nail surgery: avulsion is unnecessary. Dermatol Surg 2013;39(2):312–4.

27. Collins SC, Cordova K, Jellinek NJ. Alternatives to complete nail plate avulsion. J Am Acad Dermatol 2008;59(4):619–26.
28. Jellinek NJ. Commentary: how much is too much? Tourniquets and digital ischemia. Dermatol Surg 2013;39(4):593–5.
29. Chowdhry S, Seidenstricker L, Cooney DS, et al. Do not use epinephrine in digital blocks: myth or truth? Part II. A retrospective review of 1111 cases. Plast Reconstr Surg 2010;126(6):2031–4.
30. Denkler K. A comprehensive review of epinephrine in the finger: to do or not to do. Plast Reconstr Surg 2001;108(1):114–24.
31. Katis PG. Epinephrine in digital blocks: refuting dogma. CJEM 2003;5(4):245–6.
32. Lalonde D, Bell M, Benoit P, et al. A multicenter prospective study of 3,110 consecutive cases of elective epinephrine use in the fingers and hand: The Dalhousie Project clinical phase. J Hand Surg Am 2005;30(5):1061–7.
33. Mann T, Hammert WC. Epinephrine and hand surgery. J Hand Surg Am 2012; 37(6):1254–6 [quiz: 1257].
34. Muck AE, Bebarta VS, Borys DJ, et al. Six years of epinephrine digital injections: absence of significant local or systemic effects. Ann Emerg Med 2010;56(3): 270–4.
35. Thomson CJ, Lalonde DH, Denkler KA, et al. A critical look at the evidence for and against elective epinephrine use in the finger. Plast Reconstr Surg 2007; 119(1):260–6.
36. Harrington AC, Cheyney JM, Kinsley-Scott T, et al. A novel digital tourniquet using a sterile glove and hemostat. Dermatol Surg 2004;30(7):1065–7.
37. Lahham S, Tu K, Ni M, et al. Comparison of pressures applied by digital tourniquets in the emergency department. West J Emerg Med 2011;12(2):242–9.
38. Kain N, Koshy O. Evacuation of subungual haematomas using punch biopsy. J Plast Reconstr Aesthet Surg 2010;63(11):1932–3.
39. Telang GH, Jellinek N. Multiple calcified subungual epidermoid inclusions. J Am Acad Dermatol 2007;56(2):336–9.
40. Jellinek NJ. Nail surgery: practical tips and treatment options. Dermatol Ther 2007;20(1):68–74.
41. Baran R, Kechijian P. Hutchinson's sign: a reappraisal. J Am Acad Dermatol 1996; 34(1):87–90.
42. Kawabata Y, Ohara K, Hino H, et al. Two kinds of Hutchinson's sign, benign and malignant. J Am Acad Dermatol 2001;44(2):305–7.
43. Collins SC, Cordova KB, Jellinek NJ. Midline/paramedian longitudinal matrix excision with flap reconstruction: alternative surgical techniques for evaluation of longitudinal melanonychia. J Am Acad Dermatol 2010;62(4):627–36.
44. Haneke E. Operative Therapie akraler und subungualer Melanome. In: Rompel R, Petres J, editors. Operative und onkologische Dermatologie. Fortschritte der operativen und onkologischen Dermatologie. Berlin (Germany): Springer; 1999. p. 210–4.
45. Haneke E, Baran R. Longitudinal melanonychia. Dermatol Surg 2001;27(6): 580–4.
46. Di Chiacchio N, Loureiro WR, Michalany NS, et al. Tangential biopsy thickness versus lesion depth in longitudinal melanonychia: a pilot study. Dermatol Res Pract 2012;2012:353864.
47. Jellinek N. Nail matrix biopsy of longitudinal melanonychia: diagnostic algorithm including the matrix shave biopsy. J Am Acad Dermatol 2007;56(5):803–10.
48. Jellinek NJ. Flaps in nail surgery. Dermatol Ther 2012;25(6):535–44.

49. Jellinek NJ, Rubin AI. Lateral longitudinal excision of the nail unit. Dermatol Surg 2011;37(12):1781–5.
50. Moossavi M, Scher RK. Complications of nail surgery: a review of the literature. Dermatol Surg 2001;27(3):225–8.
51. Furukawa H, Tsutsumida A, Yamamoto Y, et al. Melanoma of thumb: retrospective study for amputation levels, surgical margin and reconstruction. J Plast Reconstr Aesthet Surg 2007;60(1):24–31.
52. Rayatt SS, Dancey AL, Davison PM. Thumb subungual melanoma: is amputation necessary? J Plast Reconstr Aesthet Surg 2007;60(6):635–8.
53. Wagner A, Garrido I, Ferron G, et al. Subungual melanoma: for a conservative approach on the thumb scale. Ann Plast Surg 2007;59(3):344–8.
54. Cohen T, Busam KJ, Patel A, et al. Subungual melanoma: management considerations. Am J Surg 2008;195(2):244–8.
55. Banfield CC, Dawber RP, Walker NP, et al. Mohs micrographic surgery for the treatment of in situ nail apparatus melanoma: a case report. J Am Acad Dermatol 1999;40(1):98–9.
56. Dika E, Piraccini BM, Balestri R, et al. Mohs surgery for squamous cell carcinoma of the nail: report of 15 cases. Our experience and a long-term follow-up. Br J Dermatol 2012;167(6):1310–4.
57. Goldminz D, Bennett RG. Mohs micrographic surgery of the nail unit. J Dermatol Surg Oncol 1992;18(8):721–6.
58. Zaiac MN, Weiss E. Mohs micrographic surgery of the nail unit and squamous cell carcinoma. Dermatol Surg 2001;27(3):246–51.
59. Jellinek NJ. Primary malignant tumors of the nail unit. Adv Dermatol 2005;21: 33–64.
60. Dika E, Fanti PA, Patrizi A, et al. Mohs surgery for squamous cell carcinoma of the nail unit: 10 years of experience. Dermatol Surg 2015;41(9):1015–9.
61. Jellinek NJ, Bauer JH. En bloc excision of the nail. Dermatol Surg 2010;36(9): 1445–50.
62. Shum C, Bruno RJ, Ristic S, et al. Examination of the anatomic relationship of the proximal germinal nail matrix to the extensor tendon insertion. J Hand Surg Am 2000;25(6):1114–7.
63. Duarte AF, Correia O, Barros AM, et al. Nail melanoma in situ: clinical, dermoscopic, pathologic clues, and steps for minimally invasive treatment. Dermatol Surg 2015;41(1):59–68.
64. Neczyporenko F, André J, Torosian K, et al. Management of in situ melanoma of the nail apparatus with functional surgery: report of 11 cases and review of the literature. J Eur Acad Dermatol Venereol 2014;28(5):550–7.
65. de Berker DA, Dahl MG, Comaish JS, et al. Nail surgery: an assessment of indications and outcome. Acta Derm Venereol 1996;76(6):484–7.
66. Richert B, Theunis A, Norrenberg S, et al. Tangential excision of pigmented nail matrix lesions responsible for longitudinal melanonychia: evaluation of the technique on a series of 30 patients. J Am Acad Dermatol 2013;69(1):96–104.
67. Ingram GJ, Scher RK, Lally EV. Reflex sympathetic dystrophy following nail biopsy. J Am Acad Dermatol 1987;16(1 Pt 2):253–6.

The Human Papillomavirus and Its Role in Plantar Warts

A Comprehensive Review of Diagnosis and Management

Tracey C. Vlahovic, DPM, FFPM RCPS (Glasg)[a],*,
M. Tariq Khan, PhD, BSc PodMed, MChS, FCPM, FFPM RCPS (Glasg)[b,c,d,e,f]

KEYWORDS

- Plantar verruca • Plantar wart • Retinoid • Candida • Marigold • Laser

KEY POINTS

- Warts are a therapeutic challenge with numerous therapies, both topical and surgical.
- They are caused by human papilloma virus (HPV) and ultimately form a benign tumor in the skin.
- HPV subtypes can cause a morphologically unique lesion on the skin.

INTRODUCTION

Viral warts or verruca pedis (plantar warts) are common skin conditions seen in both children and adults. Human papilloma virus (HPV), a DNA virus, is responsible for plantar verrucae. On the hands and feet, the HPV subtypes are typically 1, 2, 4, 27, and 57. It needs an epidermal abrasion and a transiently impaired immune system to inoculate a keratinocyte.[1]

Disclosure: T.C. Vlahovic has nothing to disclose. M.T. Khan wishes to disclose that his father pioneered marigold therapy, but he has no financial interest in the family business.
[a] Department of Podiatric Medicine, Temple University School of Podiatric Medicine, 148 North 8th Street, Philadelphia, PA 19107, USA; [b] Marigold Clinic, The Royal London Hospital for Integrated Medicine, University College London Hospital NHS Foundation Trust, 60 Great Ormond Street, London WC1N 3HR, UK; [c] Department of Dermatology, Barts Health Trust, London, UK; [d] EB Department, Great Ormond Street Hospital for Sick Children, London, UK; [e] St George Medical School, University of New South Wales, New South Wales, Australia; [f] Department of Podiatric Medicine, Temple University School of Podiatric Medicine, Philadelphia, PA, USA
* Corresponding author.
E-mail address: traceyv@temple.edu

Clin Podiatr Med Surg 33 (2016) 337–353
http://dx.doi.org/10.1016/j.cpm.2016.02.003
0891-8422/16/$ – see front matter © 2016 Elsevier Inc. All rights reserved.

Because HPV can exist on fomites, showers and swimming pools with abrasive nonslip surfaces act as high-risk areas for simultaneously harboring the virus and causing an epidermal abrasion. Thirty percent of warts may clear spontaneously, but those that do not are often cosmetically unappealing, painful, and irritating to the patient.[2] The virus seems to encourage basal cell replication. Hyperplasia of the granular and prickle cell layer occurs in addition to the dermal papillae arching its vasculature up into the wart. Keratinocytes, with an eccentric nuclei surrounded by a halo (koilocytes), show viral damage of the cells.

Plantar warts are clinically defined as well-circumscribed lesions with overlying hyperkeratosis. On debridement of the hyperkeratosis, pinpoint bleeding may be seen and interruption of the skin lines. Pain may be elicited through lateral compression of the plantar lesion, but may also be painful on ambulation with direct pressure. If it involves the nail unit, the nail may become dystrophic from the pressure and presence of the lesion.

There are several treatments for plantar verrucae; however, none of them are specific to HPV. They include nonsurgical and surgical methods, such as the use of keratolytic agents (salicylic acid), cryotherapy (liquid nitrogen), laser (pulse dye and CO_2), excision, bleomycin injections, and many folk remedies.

Human Papilloma Virus in Depth

The papillomaviruses (PVs) cause benign and malignant proliferative lesions of mucosal and cutaneous epithelia.[3] PVs are made up of 16 genera.[4] There are more than 100 HPV types that have been fully sequenced, but several HPV types that are not yet fully characterized. De Koning and colleagues[3] reported that there are 5 genera of HPV, namely alpha, beta, gamma, mu and nu and 16 species, that infect the skin.[4] HPV types belonging to species of 3 genera (alpha, gamma, and mu) have most frequently been detected in plantar warts.

The alpha-PV types infecting the genital mucosa (eg, HPV16, HPV18, HPV6, and HPV11) are the best understood. HPV16 and HPV18 are the most prevalent types involved in the pathogenesis of anogenital (eg, cervical) cancer, and HPV types 6 and 11 cause genital warts and laryngeal papillomas. The alpha-PV types belonging to species 2, 4, and 8, which have been detected in cutaneous warts, have been studied less thoroughly. At present the most frequently detected alpha-PV types in cutaneous warts are HPV types 2, 3, 10, 27, and 57.[5-13] Gamma-PV types, including HPV4, HPV60, and HPV65, have also regularly been detected in cutaneous warts.[6,7,10,14] Mu-PV types, HPV1 and HPV63, have also been detected in cutaneous warts.[15] HPV types included in the beta and nu genera have rarely been detected in cutaneous warts. Harwood and colleagues (1999) described the presence of beta-PV types in cutaneous warts of immunosuppressed patients.[8] The nu-PV genus consists of only 1 HPV type (HPV41), which was originally isolated from a facial wart.[16]

In general, cutaneous warts from immune-competent and immune-compromised patients seem to show the same genotype distributions.[11,13] This finding has to be confirmed by a large-scale study comparing the distributions in the two populations with the same techniques. The number of detected types per lesion seemed to differ between immune-competent and immunosuppressed patients.[8] At present, cutaneous warts are again the focus of attention with the increasing number of chronically immunosuppressed patients.[17,18] Significant physical and psychological morbidity in these patients may result from the existence of confluent plaques of warts present on cosmetically sensitive areas such as the face and hands and the presence of large warts occurring on pressure-bearing areas such as the feet. Although cutaneous warts constitute a highly prevalent skin condition, especially in children (33%)[19] and organ transplant recipients (45%),[20] only a few large-scale epidemiologic studies including more than 100 lesions have investigated the distribution of HPV types in cutaneous warts. These studies used different detection methods, such as general primer-mediated polymerase chain reaction (PCR) followed by HPV typing with direct sequencing[10] or by restriction enzyme cleavage of the PCR product.[12] Other methods used were multiple-type–specific PCR combined with direct sequencing,[5] in situ hybridization,[21] and (Southern) blot hybridization.[6,22,23] Although these methods are in general type specific, they are time consuming and therefore less suitable for large-scale-epidemiologic studies. In the case of multiple infections, reliable typing might also be difficult with direct sequencing of the PCR amplimer without prior molecular cloning.

De Koning and colleagues[3] evaluated a novel broad-spectrum PCR–multiplex genotyping (MPG) assay called the hyperkeratotic skin lesion (HSL) PCR/MPG for identification of established and candidate cutaneous wart HPV types. These types are included in the alpha genus species 2 (HPVs 3, 10, 28, 29, 77, and 94), species 4 (HPVs 2, 27, and 57), and species 8 (HPVs 7, 40, 43, and 91); gamma genus species 1 (HPVs 4, 65, and 95), species 2 (HPV48), species 3 (HPV50), species 4 (HPV60), and species 5 (HPV88); mu genus species 1 (HPV1) and species 2 (HPV63); and nu genus species 1 (HPV41).

Human Papilloma Virus Structure

The PVs are small nonenveloped DNA viruses that are approximately 55 nm in diameter. The genome is composed of a double strand of DNA and has 3 functional coding regions: a region for coding early viral function (E), a region for coding late viral function (L) and a long control region (LCR) that lies between them (**Fig. 1**). The diagram of HPV16 is provided to represent general HPV structure (**Table 1**).

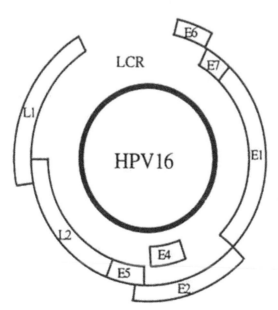

Fig. 1. HPV16 genome structure: the coding regions are represented by open boxes. (*From* Phillips AC, Vousden KH. Analysis of the interaction between human papillomavirus type 16 E7 and the TATA binding protein TBP. J Gen Virol 1997;78:905–9; with permission.)

Table 1
HPV16 structure

Gene/Region	Function
E1/E2	Codes for proteins that control the function of E6 and E7 genes
E4	Function largely unknown but may control virus release from cell
E5	Codes for a hydrophobic protein that enhances immortalization of the cell
E6	Codes for proteins that inhibit negative regulators of the cell cycle. E6 products inhibit p53, which is a transcription factor for apoptosis (programmed cell death)
E7	Codes for products that bind to the retinoblastoma tumor suppressor proteins, thereby permitting the cell to progress through the cell cycle in the absence of normal mitogenic signals
L1/L2	Codes for structural proteins and formation of complete virus particles. LCR necessary for normal virus replication and control of gene expression

PATIENT EVALUATION OVERVIEW
Clinical Manifestations of Human Papilloma Virus Infection

PV enters the body when trauma or damage to the skin occurs, leading to a portal for the virus to enter and invade to the third layer of the skin, known as the stratum spinosum. Viral DNA synthesis and virion production are probably related to the sequence of keratinocyte differentiation. These events are poorly understood, but in essence it is thought the genome is only minimally expressed in the basal cells, whereas viral DNA and capsid synthesis and assembly occur in the upper layers of the stratum spinosum and granulosum, with the virions probably being shed in the stratum corneum.[24] The virus then embeds within the surrounding papillaries, and it is often not detectable by the body's natural defenses. It can take up to 12 months for the verruca/wart to appear.[24]

The HPV subtype can be identified by the appearance of the verruca/wart for diagnosis:

- Common warts (HPVs 2, 4, 7, 26–29, and 57) can appear as small, flesh-colored papules that are dome shaped, rough, irregular, or hyperkeratotic, or they may appear as raised papillaries. They can present as mosaic, filiform, endophytic, and butcher's warts and can be found on the feet, hands, fingers, genitals, and lips.
- Myrmecia warts (HPV1) are painful palmar and plantar warts. They appear as a rough, horny surface projecting slightly above the skin, surrounded by a horny collar. Myrmecia warts usually occur singly, but they can also be multiple. They are common in children aged 5 to 15 years, and present on the palms, soles, fingers, toes, and under the nails, but rarely on the face, scalp, or body (**Figs. 2** and **3**).
- Mosaic warts (HPV2) present on the soles as a superficial, slightly raised, hyperkeratotic plaque consisting of several small warts that appear confluent with polygonal outlines. They are generally painless, and are notorious for their longevity and resistance to treatment (**Fig. 4**).
- Filiform warts (HPV3) present on orifices and the face and beard regions. Size varies from 10 nm to a few millimeters. They appear confluent, hypertrophic, and periungual, and are grey, brown, or flesh colored (**Fig. 5**).
- Endophytic warts (HPV4) present on either palmar or plantar areas. They are small punctate lesions, with a horny wall surrounding a central depression. These

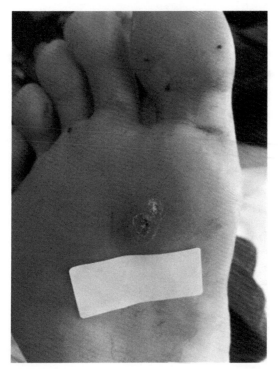

Fig. 2. Myrmecia wart.

warts occur in groups and are painless. They are often misdiagnosed as myrmecia (HPV1); however, endophytic warts have a hard keratin mass, in contrast with a soft keratin mass in myrmecia (**Fig. 6**).

- Butcher's warts (HPV7), which are seen frequently in people who work with meat, appear as large, cauliflowerlike, proliferative warts occurring on the hands and toes. They can coexist with other types of common warts (**Fig. 7**).

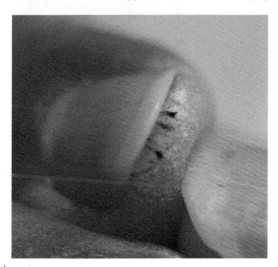

Fig. 3. Subungual wart.

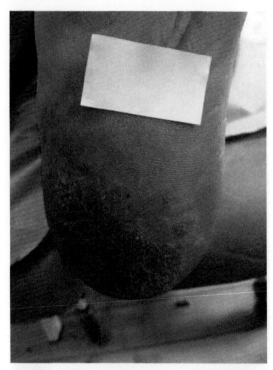

Fig. 4. Mosaic wart.

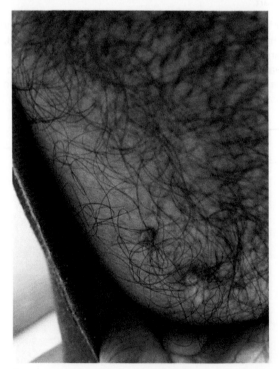

Fig. 5. Filiform wart.

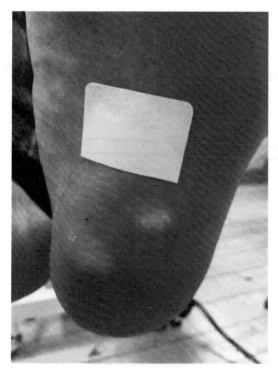

Fig. 6. Endophytic wart.

- Flat warts, also called plane warts (HPVs 3, 10, 27–29, 41) are raised warts, smaller than common warts, with flatter, smoother surfaces and irregular outlines. They occur in multiples, ranging from 2 to several hundreds and are irregular, disseminated, or grouped and confluent. These warts are localized to the face and dorsum of the hands. On the face they appear flat and pigmented, and on the hands they are elevated. Commonly seen in children, young women, and immunocompromised patients, they can resolve spontaneously.

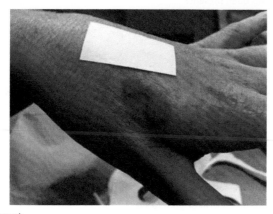

Fig. 7. Butcher's wart.

- Genital warts (HPVs 16 and 18) are generally found to be sexually transmitted and they can progress to penile, cervical, and vulvar cancers.

Plantar verrucae/warts have a limited time of existence; the average life cycle of the virus is up to 2 years. From 65% to 78% of verrucae disappear spontaneously without treatment.[2] In children, 50%[2] of verrucae regress within 6 months. Persistent verrucae/warts that are present for more than 2 years are classed as recalcitrant. They are most often seen in individuals who are immunosuppressed, such as transplant patients. This presentation is generally caused by the medication that is being taken; for example, cyclosporine or azathioprine. These types of verrucae/warts often remain for several years. Patients who have had previous plantar warts have a higher risk than those who have never had a wart.[25,26]

Evaluation of Patients with Plantar Warts

Patients seek treatment of their plantar verrucae because of embarrassment or pain.[25] Because the patient's immune status plays a role in wart development, it is important to assess the past and current immune state. A thorough history and physical takes into consideration the questions in **Box 1** and a visual inspection to determine the type of wart present (discussed earlier). Plantar warts can either be nonpainful or painful depending on their anatomic location and sensitivity of the patient. The various presentations on the lower extremity, including the flesh-colored endophytic plantar wart, the periungual lesion, the mosaic wart, and a filiform cutaneous hornlike lesion, create a challenge for diagnosis and management. Differential diagnoses include pitted keratolysis, punctate keratosis, corn, callus, molluscum contagiosum, and squamous cell carcinoma (particularly the subtype verrucous carcinoma).[25]

Plantar warts are commonly flesh-colored, discreet lesions that may occur singly or in multiples. A confluence of these lesions appears as a mosaic pattern. Lesions may occur in non–weight-bearing areas or in weight-bearing areas. Pain on lateral compression may assist in diagnosis, but patients may report pain on direct compression caused by ambulation. One of the most common signs that a plantar verruca is present is the interruption of the dermal glyphics on the foot. This interruption of the skin lines can be seen with the naked eye, but is enhanced when viewing with a

---

Box 1
Questions to ask patients with plantar warts

1. How long has this been present?
2. Is it painful?
3. Which lesion presented first?
4. Do you have sweaty feet?
5. What over-the-counter or home remedies have you tried?
6. If you have been treated by another physician or have tried yourself, did the treatment provided cause the warts to get smaller, larger, or not change? Were they ever cut out at some point?
7. Have you picked at them? If you have, did they get larger?
8. Do you have warts anywhere else on the body (eg, fingers, face, knees)?
9. Does anyone else in your family have warts or do you share space with someone who does (eg, a grandchild who visits)? Do you share shoes with anyone?
10. Do you go barefoot at a gym or pool facility?

dermatoscope. Following the reappearance of the skin lines throughout the lesion aids clinicians in determining resolution of the lesion.

Asking about hyperhidrosis, picking of lesions, and worsening of the lesion after previous treatments allows clinicians to determine whether the Koebner phenomenon is occurring. The Koebner phenomenon or isomorphic response is the development of pathologic lesions in traumatized uninvolved skin, which can occur during treatment of a verruca.[25] Many clinicians associate this response with psoriatic lesions, but it also occurs in Kaposi sarcoma, lichen planus, and warts caused by HPV.[25] After trauma to the skin, new lesions arise that are histopathologically identical to the original lesion. Many patients report having a small lesion at the first physician visit, consenting to the procedure that they thought would be curative, and only then to having multiple and sometimes larger lesions return a few weeks to months after the procedure. This outcome causes frustration for both the clinician and patient. It is important to keep this phenomenon in mind when choosing the treatment plan, especially in a patient who has failed excision of the lesion. Ultimately clearance of the lesion is based on the patient's immune status, the HPV type present and its reaction to the therapy applied, and the extent and longevity of the warts.[25]

CLINICAL MANAGEMENT OF VERRUCA PEDIS
Pharmacologic and Nonpharmacologic Treatment Options

Therapeutic options are intended to eliminate the signs and symptoms of the wart because there is no cure for HPV. Not all therapies work on all patients, and often 2 or more have to be combined on the patient's foot to produce a clinical change. An ideal wart therapy is painless, resolves most or all lesions, offers no scarring after treatment, involves 1 to 3 office visits, and offers lifetime HPV immunity.[25] Also, because randomized controlled clinical trial evidence is lacking, the literature shows anecdotal, small case series that all seem to have an effect.

Because no single treatment technique and no specific antiviral therapy have been developed, plantar warts are a therapeutic challenge for both clinicians and patients. Different modalities described in the literature range from tissue keratolysis (salicylic acid) to immunotherapy (bleomycin) to tissue destructive (cryotherapy, surgical excision).[25] Eradication of verruca pedis/plantar warts ultimately is based on the activation of the body's immune system to fight the virus. Many treatment options are available, with differing success rates. Clinicians may choose therapy based on cost, pain induction, and other side effects that work with the patient's occupation and/or lifestyle.

Unique to plantar verrucae, sharp debridement of the lesion is necessary to remove the hyperkeratotic covering in order to improve topical therapy penetration and provide symptomatic pain relief. This debridement is performed before most therapies done in office. Pinpoint bleeding often occurs on debridement. This bleeding should be avoided if a nonablative laser (ie, pulsed dye or yttrium-aluminum-garnet [YAG]) is to be applied to the lesion. The target chromophore for these devices is oxyhemoglobin, and, if blood is present on the surface, the laser's target may be too superficial to have a therapeutic effect.

Folk remedies

Numerous folk remedies have been described that use fruit (rubbing a banana), a vegetable plus the right environment (performing a ritual with a potato during the full moon and then burying it), and animals (rubbing a toad on the wart). However outlandish these might seem, it is important to realize that because most warts have a finite presence, these remedies may coincide with the wart's spontaneous resolution.

Salicylic acid

Salicylic acid, a keratolytic that lyses the epidermis, is the first-line therapy chosen by many clinicians to perform in office (compounded up to 60% strength), but is also what the patient may unwillingly choose when faced with the over-the-counter options (17% or 40% preparations).[25] After debridement, the clinician applies the salicylic acid to an aperture pad followed by occlusive tape. The patient has to keep the area dry for 5 to 7 days. In contrast, the over-the-counter preparations require daily or every-other-day application of the salicylic acid preparation. Both home and in-office therapy may require multiple treatments, but, from a retrospective review of evidence-based data, this has an effectiveness of about 75%.[27] Because it is cost-effective and not often painful, it presents as an effective initial therapy for many patients.

Cryotherapy

Another in-office first-line therapy performed by clinicians is cryotherapy, or the application of liquid nitrogen directly to the verruca. This therapy is generally painful and causes a cell-mediated response via local inflammation, but does not kill the virus directly. The newly available over-the-counter cryotherapies are not as cold as liquid nitrogen. Like liquid nitrogen, the over-the-counter version may cause hypopigmentation; blistering; a ring wart, or a circular resurgence of the wart around where the skin was frozen (a Koebner response); and pain. In general, the cryogen is applied to the wart until a white halo appears (ie, freezing of the skin) once every 2 weeks. Because differences in technique can vary in the literature, cure rates range from 39% to 92%.[25] A more aggressive technique may yield better results but also lead to more adverse events experienced by the patient. This therapy can also be used in combination with other modalities, like salicylic acid.

Topical retinoids

Topical retinoids are commonly used for acne; they alter keratinization in the epidermis, act as an antiinflammatory, and inhibit cell proliferation. Although adapalene 0.1% gel is used in the treatment of mild to moderate acne, a current article in the *Indian Journal of Dermatology* described its use for plantar verrucae.[28] Fifty patients who had 424 plantar warts were randomized into either group A (adapalene 0.1% gel under occlusion) or group B (cryotherapy). Group A applied adapalene 0.1% twice daily under occlusion and group B received cryotherapy once every 2 weeks. Patients were followed weekly until warts cleared and then reported for monthly visits for 6 months postclearance to determine whether there was any recurrence.

Twenty-four out of 25 patients in group A had complete clearance of 286 warts in about 36 days. Group B's cryotherapy treatments had 24 out of 25 patients develop complete clearance of 124 warts in 52 days. Group A patients experienced no adverse events, whereas group B had scarring, pain, and redness (all the side effects that are expected with the use of cryotherapy). There was no recurrence in any patient. In this study, adapalene 0.1% gel seemed to clear warts faster and with fewer side effects than cryotherapy alone. This treatment is an off-label indication for plantar verrucae based on a single study.

Topical 5-fluorouracil

Topical 5-fluorouracil (5-FU) is used primarily to treat actinic keratosis on the body. It has been used off-label for warts because it is thought that it inhibits cellular proliferation.[29] In a prospective, randomized controlled study, Salk and colleagues[29] compared topical 5-FU application under tape occlusion versus tape occlusion alone.

Nineteen out of 20 patients in the 5-FU/tape arm had complete resolution after 12 weeks of treatment. A few had recurrence 6 months later, but overall most patients retained their verruca-free state.

Cimetidine

Cimetidine, an H2-receptor antagonist, has been shown to exert inhibition of the suppressor T-cell function at its histamine 2 receptor site.[30] Originally shown to assist with recalcitrant warts in children, the treatment regimen was extrapolated for use in adults with daily doses of 20 to 40 mg/kg.[30] Open-label studies showed promise, but small randomized controlled trials showed no difference between the drug and placebo.[25] In an 8-year retrospective study, patients (aged 3–25+ years) who had received cimetidine as monotherapy or after failing other treatments were reviewed.[30] Across all age groups, treatment success was 84.3%, with 86% in the pediatric group and 75.8% in the adult group. Adults had 4 times the recurrence rate of the children in the study. Because cimetidine seems to be a safe option, its efficacy rate across the literature is variable, making its success difficult to distinguish from a placebolike effect.

Duct tape

In an article by Focht and colleagues,[31] the practice of using duct tape to treat plantar warts increased in popularity among both clinicians and lay people alike. Having warts on all parts of the body, 61 patients aged 3 to 22 years received either cryotherapy (liquid nitrogen) treatment every 2 to 3 weeks (for up to 6 sessions) or duct tape application once every 6 days for up to 2 months. Eighty-five percent of the warts resolved in the duct tape arm versus 60% in the cryotherapy arm. The mechanism of action remains unclear, but may relate to local irritation caused by the adhesive or the act of occlusion that duct tape causes. However, in the study it was difficult for the patients with plantar warts to keep the tape on consistently because of hyperhidrosis and shoe gear. Although this may be a cost-effective therapy for patients who are unwilling or unable to see a physician, more research is needed to determine the true efficacy in plantar verrucae.

Cantharidin

Cantharidin, a blistering agent, is derived from the beetle, *Cantharis vesicatoria*.[25] It is not currently available in the United States, but can be purchased from other countries. After debridement, a thin layer of cantharidin (also available in a compounded formula with podophyllin and salicylic acid) is applied to the wart and covered with occlusive tape. The area is washed with soap and water after between 6 and 24 hours, and a possible blister may form. This process is repeated once every 2 weeks. It is nonpainful to apply, but may be fairly disabling when the blister forms. Literature reports cure rates as high as 80%, but there are no randomized controlled studies using cantharidin on plantar warts.[25]

Bleomycin

Bleomycin, a potent DNA and protein synthesis inhibitor, is used as a chemotherapeutic agent that has antiviral, antibacterial, and antitumor properties.[32] It is reserved as therapy for recalcitrant warts.[25] It causes tissue necrosis that elicits an immune response and should not be used in pregnant or breast-feeding women, children, immunosuppressed patients, or vascularly compromised patients. If injected without a lidocaine mixture or block, it is extremely painful on injection. Within a day, a black ecchymotic eschar may form.

In a placebo-controlled study of palmoplantar warts (bleomycin vs saline solution), a 15-mg bottle of bleomycin powder was reconstituted with 5 mL of saline and kept as stock solution. This solution was then prepared with 2 parts of 2% lidocaine and 1 part of stock solution in a tuberculin syringe. After debridement, the solution was injected intralesionally in increments depending on the size of the lesion. This process was repeated in 2 weeks if necessary and patients were followed for a year. After 1 or 2 injections, 96.15% of the palmoplantar warts responded.[32]

For patients who wish to avoid injection, another technique of applying the bleomycin solution by dropping it on a debrided wart has been described. This technique showed a 92% clearance rate.[33] Bleomycin has high rates of effectiveness, but may not be the ideal therapy for every patient.

Candida immunotherapy

Injection of *Candida albicans* skin test allergen has been described in the literature as a therapeutic option for plantar warts.[34] Previous articles have shown that injection of a site on the foot often clears distant wart sites like the hands or knees.[35] Vlahovic and colleagues[36] performed a retrospective review of 80 patients who were injected with *C albicans* skin test allergen in the primary or largest plantar verruca (Nielsen biosciences, San Diego, CA), and 65% had a successful treatment (skin lines returned to lesion). Patients who were in the failure group either were lost to follow-up or did not meet the criteria of having skin lines return throughout the lesion. When examining the data further, it was determined that 4 visits occurred to clear the lesion (consistent with the literature), and that patients who had had a previous tissue-destructive procedure (cantharidin, salicylic acid, various lasers) before initiating the *Candida* regimen were almost 3 times more likely to clear once injection therapy was started than those who had no previous therapy and began with the *Candida* injection process. Most likely this shows that warts need a multimodal approach to resolve.

Phytotherapy

Phytotherapy, or the application of a plant-based material to the skin, has been used for centuries for various ailments. The use of plants to treat warts is not new (eg, folk remedies), but 1 plant in particular has been studied: the marigold. Marigold therapy was first described in the podiatric literature as a treatment of plantar hyperkeratotic lesions in 1980.[37] Marigold therapy involves the use of a marigold paste in alcohol that is placed directly on the plantar wart in an offloading pad for 5 to 7 days. The *Tagetes* genus of marigold has been found to be strongly keratolytic. The keratolytic and anti-inflammatory properties of *Tagetes* in the treatment of verrucae and hyperkeratotic lesions have been well documented in the literature.[38,39] In one study, 40 patients were randomly placed into one of 4 groups; active, placebo, active with offloading felt pad, and pad only with no paste.[39] Patients were treated twice a week for 2 weeks with the marigold paste and then used a marigold-based home therapy program. The lesion surface area pretreatment and posttreatment was analyzed with a wound mapping system. Results showed that the active group had a significant difference in appearance, pain, and size compared with the placebo group.

It has been reported that the chemicals found in the multiple *Tagetes* species have a proposed method of action as an antiviral: cellular apoptosis of the HPV-infected keratinocyte. Studies have shown this is a noninvasive and painless therapy, and further research will assess the effectiveness of this as monotherapy and as an adjunct to other modalities.

An additional phytotherapeutic agent, *Thuja occidentalis*, a member of the conifer tree family, had its proposed antiviral properties studied using 30 randomly selected patients.[40,41] Patients were chosen with lesions older than 18 months. An extract containing *T occidentalis* was applied daily for 3 weeks and followed for 6 months after initial treatment. Ninety percent of patients had resolution of their lesions after 1 month from the initial treatment. At 6 months, the same number of patients had no recurrence. After the assessment, a double-blind placebo-controlled study showed that 80% of the active group had resolution, whereas the placebo group had just 33% resolution.[41]

Human papilloma virus vaccine

Both Gardasil (HPV quadrivalent [types 6, 11, 16, 18] vaccine, recombinant) and Cervarix (HPV bivalent [types 16 and 18] vaccine, recombinant) are HPV vaccines that are intended to decrease the incidence of cervical cancer by preventing infection by certain HPV types. Gardasil is given to both male and female patients in a series of 3 injections: baseline, 2 months, and 6 months. With the recent evidence that Gardasil protects male as well as female patients equally from developing genital warts, it seems that the age range of 9 to 26 years will be receiving the vaccination more than ever before.[42] This development leads to the question: will this be helpful in eradicating current, or preventing future, plantar verrucae in this population?

Because there have been no clinical trials to address the use of the vaccines for verruca vulgaris and plantar verruca, there is only anecdotal evidence. In observations during the Gardasil clinical trials, the investigators noted that patients who already had both verruca vulgaris and plantar verruca before their vaccination had some warts clear during the trial. It was also noted that Gardasil had a protective effect against neoplasia in subjects who had HPV types 1, 2, and 3.[43] Most plantar warts are caused by HPV types 1, 2, 4, or 63; these types are not targeted by either of the vaccines, which target the strains that are the highest risk for transformation of an HPV infection into malignancy.

Because evidence of Gardasil's cross-protection with related HPV strains[31,44,45] has been shown, plus the anecdotal evidence discussed earlier, it is no surprise that 2 articles in *Archives of Dermatology* reported significant reduction of palmar and plantar verruca.[46] In a 31-year-old man with a history of epilepsy and developmental delay, more than 30 warts on his hands (and some on the feet) cleared after administration of the 3 Gardasil injections and there was no recurrence 18 months after the initial injection.[43] The HPV type of this patient's warts was not identified, but he had no previous history of genital warts or other significant history. In another case, a 41-year-old woman with a 10-year history of both palmoplantar warts and WILD syndrome (disseminated warts, depressed cellular mediated immunity, primary lymphedema, and anogenital dysplasia) tested positive for HPV type 57 in her cutaneous warts.[44] Four weeks after the initial administration of Gardasil, the patient's warts significantly reduced. Six months after the last injection, most of the palmoplantar warts had substantially improved or even cleared. Other case series have shown anecdotal success with warts in multiple locations, including the feet.[47] Because this is a common vaccination in teenagers, it is important for practicing clinicians to note any changes that may occur when an adolescent with plantar warts is subject to this injection.

LASER

One of the first lasers to be used on plantar verrucae, the carbon dioxide (CO_2) laser, is an ablative laser in the infrared spectrum whose beam acts as a scalpel.[48] Its beam targets water and is nonselective in its tissue destruction. Even though it leaves a cauterized and clean surgical field, the area targeted must heal by secondary intention. When performing this procedure on a patient, it is important for the clinician to discuss the possibility of scar, delayed healing, and postoperative pain. It is suggested to wear a mask, have a smoke evacuator, and take other precautions because of the plume that this laser creates.[49] There have been no randomized controlled studies using just the CO_2 laser, but there have been reports of its use combined with topical therapies like imiquimod 5% cream, which show moderate success.[50]

The neodymium YAG (Nd:YAG) laser has a wavelength of 1064 nm, which is also in the infrared range. However, this is a nonablative laser whose target chromophore (the entity in the body that absorbs the laser wavelength) is oxyhemoglobin, which allows selective heating of the capillary-rich active verrucae.[51] The nonablative pulsed dye laser (PDL) also targets oxyhemoglobin around the 585-nm to 595-nm wavelength.[51] In a study following 46 patients, warts were either treated with the Nd:YAG or the PDL. Because the Nd:YAG wavelength is absorbed less well than the pulsed dye wavelength by oxyhemoglobin, a higher fluence (energy per surface area) is needed and applied for the Nd:YAG versus the PDL.[52] The Nd:YAG was applied at a fluence of 100 J/cm^2 compared with the pulsed dye fluence of 8 J/cm^2. There was no significant difference in the use of the two lasers (clearance rates of 73.9% PDL vs 78.3% Nd:YAG) except the Nd:YAG was more painful and the PDL required more treatments. This observation is consistent with what the first author (TV) has seen in patients receiving laser therapy. Both lasers produce less downtime and possible scarring than the CO_2 device.

SURGICAL TREATMENT OPTIONS

Excision of the verruca is commonly practiced. It can involve sole excochleation of the lesion, curettage followed by cauterization, or a true excisional procedure. No randomized controlled studies have been published using this technique for the foot. Because success rates of 65% to 85% have been reported, the most problematic sequelae of these procedures are scarring and recurrence.[25] Both can occur in up to 30% of patients.[45,53] Recurrence has been attributed to activation of the Koebner phenomenon where the latent virus next to the original wart becomes active.[54] A recurring wart within a scar is a challenging entity to manage and often results in frustration for practitioners and patients. From an anatomic and pain perspective, scarring can be particularly problematic on plantar feet, so this technique is best practiced for warts on the limbs and face. Excision of plantar warts is not recommended as a standard, first-line therapy because of pain, likely recurrence, and resulting plantar scar.[55]

SUMMARY/DISCUSSION

HPV infection of the skin is a fascinating and complex disease entity that creates a therapeutic conundrum for both patients and physicians. Treatment of these lesions requires consideration of the host's immune status, the type of HPV involved, the anatomic location, and the tolerance for a certain procedure from a lifestyle perspective. The goal of therapy is to destroy the lesion in the fewest visits with the least pain. At this time, there is no single therapy to provide painless wart destruction in 1 visit, but a combination of the treatments discussed in this article is most likely to result in a positive therapeutic outcome.

REFERENCES

1. Vlahovic TC, Schleicher SM. Skin disease of the lower extremities: a photographic guide. HMP Communications; 2012.

2. Sterling JC, Handfield-Jones S, Hudson PM, British Association of Dermatologists. Guidelines for management of cutaneous warts. Br J Dermatol 2001; 144(1):4–11.

3. de Koning MN, ter Schegget J, Eekhof JA, et al. Evaluation of a novel broad-spectrum PCR-multiplex genotyping assay for identification of cutaneous wart-associated human papillomavirus types. J Clin Microbiol 2010;48(5):1706–11.
4. de Villiers EM, Fauquet C, Broker TR, et al. Classification of papillomaviruses. Virology 2004;324:17–27.
5. Chan SY, Chew SH, Egawa K, et al. Phylogenetic analysis of the human papillomavirus type 2 (HPV-2), HPV-27, and HPV-57 group, which is associated with common warts. Virology 1997;239:296–302.
6. Gassenmaier A, Fuchs P, Schell H, et al. Papillomavirus DNA in warts of immunosuppressed renal allograft recipients. Arch Dermatol Res 1986;278:219–23.
7. Hagiwara K, Uezato H, Arakaki H, et al. A genotype distribution of human papillomaviruses detected by polymerase chain reaction and direct sequencing analysis in a large sample of common warts in Japan. J Med Virol 2005;77:107–12.
8. Harwood CA, Spink PJ, Surentheran T, et al. Degenerate and nested PCR: a highly sensitive and specific method for detection of human papillomavirus infection in cutaneous warts. J Clin Microbiol 1999;37:3545–55.
9. Lai JY, Doyle RJ, Bluhm JM, et al. Multiplexed PCR genotyping of HPVs from plantaris verrucae. J Clin Virol 2006;35:435–41.
10. Pfister H. Chapter 8: human papillomavirus and skin cancer. J Natl Cancer Inst Monogr 2003;31:52–6.
11. Porro AM, Alchorne MM, Mota GR, et al. Detection and typing of human papillomavirus in cutaneous warts of patients infected with human immunodeficiency virus type 1. Br J Dermatol 2003;149:1192–9.
12. Rübben A, Kalka K, Spelten B, et al. Clinical features and age distribution of patients with HPV 2/27/57-induced common warts. Arch Dermatol Res 1997;289:337–40.
13. Rübben A, Krones R, Schwetschenau R, et al. Common warts from immunocompetent patients show the same distribution of human papillomavirus types as common warts from immunocompromised patients. Br J Dermatol 1993;128:264–70.
14. Chen SL, Tsao YP, Lee JW, et al. Characterization and analysis of human papillomaviruses of skin warts. Arch Dermatol Res 1993;285:460–5.
15. Egawa K, Delius H, Matsukura T, et al. Two novel types of human papillomavirus, HPV 63 and HPV 65: comparisons of their clinical and histological features and DNA sequences to other HPV types. Virology 1993;194:789–99.
16. Grimmel M, de Villiers EM, Neumann C, et al. Characterization of a new human papillomavirus (HPV 41) from disseminated warts and detection of its DNA in some skin carcinomas. Int J Cancer 1988;41:5–9.
17. Euvrard S, Kanitakis J, Claudy A. Skin cancers after organ transplantation. N Engl J Med 2003;348:1681–91.
18. Ulrich C, Hackethal M, Meyer T, et al. Skin infections in organ transplant recipients. J Dtsch Dermatol Ges 2008;6:98–105.
19. van Haalen FM, Bruggink SC, Gussekloo J, et al. Warts in primary schoolchildren: prevalence and relation with environmental factors. Br J Dermatol 2009;161:148–52.
20. Bouwes Bavinck JN, Euvrard S, Naldi L, et al. Keratotic skin lesions and other risk factors are associated with skin cancer in organ-transplant recipients: a case-control study in The Netherlands, United Kingdom, Germany, France, and Italy. J Invest Dermatol 2007;127:1647–56.

21. Egawa K, Honda Y, Inaba Y, et al. Pigmented viral warts: a clinical and histopathological study including human papillomavirus typing. Br J Dermatol 1998;138: 381–9.

22. Egawa K. New types of human papillomaviruses and intracytoplasmic inclusion bodies: a classification of inclusion warts according to clinical features, histology and associated HPV types. Br J Dermatol 1994;130:158–66.

23. Phillips AC, Vousden KH. Analysis of the interaction between human papillomavirus type 16 E7 and the TATA binding protein TBP. J Gen Virol 1997;78:905–9.

24. Bernard HU. Controls in the papillomavirus life cycle. FEMS Microbiol Immunol 1990;2(4):201–5.

25. Lipke MM. An armamentarium of wart treatments. Clin Med Res 2006;4(4): 273–93.

26. Thappa DM. The isomorphic phenomenon of Koebner. Indian J Dermatol Venereol Leprol 2004;70:187–9. Available at: http://www.ijdvl.com/text.asp?2004/70/3/187/11105. Accessed November 30, 2015.

27. Gibbs S, Harvey I, Sterling JC, et al. Local treatments for cutaneous warts. Cochrane Database Syst Rev 2003;(3):CD001781.

28. Gupta R, Gupta S. Topical adapalene in the treatment of plantar warts; randomized comparative open trial in comparison with cryo-therapy. Indian J Dermatol 2015;60(1):102.

29. Salk RS, Grogan KA, Chang TJ. Topical 5% 5-fluorouracil cream in the treatment of plantar warts: a prospective, randomized, and controlled clinical study. J Drugs Dermatol 2006;5(5):418–24.

30. Mullen BR, Guiliana JV, Nesheiwat F. Cimetidine as a first-line therapy for pedal verruca. J Am Podiatr Med Assoc 2005;95(3):229–34.

31. Focht DR 3rd, Spicer C, Fairchok MP. The efficacy of duct tape vs cryotherapy in the treatment of verruca vulgaris (the common wart). Arch Pediatr Adolesc Med 2002;156:971–4.

32. Soni P, Khandelwal K, Aara N, et al. Efficacy of intralesional bleomycin in palmoplantar and periungual warts. J Cutan Aesthet Surg 2011;4(3):188–91.

33. Munn SE, Higgins E, Marshall M, et al. A new method of intralesional bleomycin therapy in the treatment of recalcitrant warts. Br J Dermatol 1996;135:969–71.

34. Signore RJ. *Candida albicans* intralesional injection immunotherapy of warts. Cutis 2002;70:185.

35. Clifton MM, Johnson SM, Roberson PK, et al. Immunotherapy for recalcitrant warts in children using intralesional mumps or *Candida* antigens. Pediatr Dermatol 2003;20:268.

36. Vlahovic TC, Spadone S, Dunn SP, et al. *Candida albicans* immunotherapy for verrucae plantaris. J Am Podiatr Med Assoc 2015;105(5):395–400.

37. Davidson L. Marigold rediscovered: a cure for callosities. Therapy 1980;1.

38. Khan MT Jr. *Tagetes signata* in the treatment of verruca pedis. J British Pod Med 1996;51:118b.

39. Khan MT, Khan MT. A double blind placebo study of topical *Tagetes* on verruca pedis in children and adults. J Eur Acad Dermatol Venereol 1999;1:S251.

40. Khan MT, Cerio R, Khan MT Sr. The efficacy of *Thuja occidentalis* on verruca pedis in children and adults. J Eur Acad Dermatol Venereol 1998;11:S150.

41. Khan MT, Cerio R, Watt R, et al. A double blind placebo study of topical *Thuja occidentalis* on verruca pedis in children and adults. J Eur Acad Dermatol Venereol 1999;1:S251.

42. Available at: http://healthland.time.com/2011/02/03/gardasil-protects-boys-and-men-from-hpv-too/. Accessed March 18, 2016.

43. Venugopal SS, Murrell DF. Recalcitrant cutaneous warts treated with recombinant quadrivalent human papillomavirus vaccine (types 6, 11, 16, and 18) in a developmentally delayed, 31-year-old white man. Arch Dermatol 2010;146(5):475–7.

44. Kreuter A, Waterboer T, Wieland U. Regression of cutaneous warts in a patient with WILD syndrome following recombinant quadrivalent human papillomavirus vaccination. Arch Dermatol 2010;146(10):1196–7.

45. Pringle WM, Helms DC. Treatment of plantar warts by blunt dissection. Arch Dermatol 1973;108:79–82.

46. Ault KA. Human papillomavirus vaccines and the potential for cross-protection between related HPV types. Gynecol Oncol 2007;107(2 Suppl 1):S31–3.

47. Daniel BS, Murrell DF. Complete resolution of chronic multiple verruca vulgaris treated with quadrivalent human papillomavirus vaccine. JAMA Dermatol 2013; 149(3):370–2.

48. Serour F, Somekh E. Successful treatment of recalcitrant warts in pediatric patients with carbon dioxide laser. Eur J Pediatr Surg 2003;13:219–23.

49. Gloster HM, Roenigk R. Risk of acquiring human papillomavirus from the plume produced by the carbon dioxide laser in the treatment of warts. J Am Acad Dermatol 1995;32(3):436–41.

50. Zeng Y, Zheng Y, Wang L. Vagarious successful treatment of recalcitrant warts in combination with CO_2 laser and imiquimod 5% cream. J Cosmet Laser Ther 2014;16(6):311–3.

51. Patil UA, Dhami LD. Overview of lasers. Indian J Plast Surg 2008;41(Suppl): S101–13.

52. El-Mohamady Ael-S, Mearag I, El-Khalawany M, et al. Pulsed dye laser versus Nd:YAG laser in the treatment of plantar warts: a comparative study. Lasers Med Sci 2014;29(3):1111–6.

53. Baruch K. Blunt dissection for the treatment of plantar verrucae. Cutis 1990;46: 145–7, 151-2.

54. Leman JA, Benton EC. Verrucas. Guidelines for management. Am J Clin Dermatol 2000;1:143–9.

55. Arndt KA, Bowers KE, Alam M, et al. Warts. In: Manual of dermatologic therapeutics. 6th edition. Philadelphia: Lippincott Williams & Wilkins; 2002. p. 241–51.

Psoriasis

Pathogenesis, Assessment, and Therapeutic Update

Stephen M. Schleicher, MD[a,b,c,d],*

KEYWORDS

- Psoriasis • Biologics • Psoriatic comorbidities • Psoriatic arthritis

KEY POINTS

- Psoriasis is a chronic condition that affects more than 7 million Americans.
- The disorder has no known cure but today an overwhelming majority of patients can achieve good to excellent control.
- Over the past 2 decades, enhanced understanding of the immunologic basis of psoriasis has led to the development of new systemic agents that have revolutionized the management of this disease.
- There are significant barriers to optimal management, which include expense, patient compliance, and medication safety.
- When dealing with this disease, health care providers should strive to identify the most efficacious treatment associated with the fewest possible adverse events delivered at a reasonable cost.

Psoriasis is a chronic immune-mediated inflammatory disease that affects more than 7 million Americans and 2% to 4% of the population worldwide.[1–3] Affected individuals are impacted both psychologically and physically. Patients with psoriasis are at increased risk of developing anxiety and depression[4] as well as cardiometabolic and rheumatologic comorbidities, all of which can greatly reduce quality of life.[5] Most patients with psoriasis require chronic care, and disease-associated therapeutic management costs billions of dollars on an annual basis in the United States.[6]

Financial Disclosure: Dr S.M. Schleicher is a speaker for Aqua Pharmaceuticals and Celgene and has served as a Principal Investigator for Amgen, Exeltis, Galderma, Genentech, Regeneron, and Taro.

[a] DermDOX Center for Dermatology, 20 North Laurel Street, Hazleton, PA 18201, USA; [b] St. Luke's Health Systems, 801 Ostrum Street, Bethlehem, PA 18015, USA; [c] The Commonwealth Medical College, Scranton, PA 18605, USA; [d] University of Pennsylvania Medical College, Philadelphia, PA 19104, USA
* DermDOX Center for Dermatology, 20 North Laurel Street, Hazleton, PA 18201.
E-mail address: sschleicher@dermdox.org

PATHOGENESIS

Psoriasis in predisposed individuals can be triggered by several factors, including infection, medications, and trauma (also known as the Koebner effect). Research over the past 2 decades confirms that psoriasis is a disorder resulting from immune dysregulation.[7] A complex relationship involving macrophages, dendritic cells, T cells, and cytokines induce many of the pathologic changes associated with this disease. Activated cells produce mediators of inflammation, such as tumor necrosis factor (TNF) and interleukins (ILs) 17 and 23, and it is this inflammatory response that eventuates in the skin and joint disease. Understanding the immunologic basis of psoriasis has led to the development of new therapies and a revolutionary approach to management.

GENETICS

Psoriasis has a significant genetic predisposition, with elevated incidence in first-degree and second-degree relatives.[8] Incidence is equal in men and women. In the United States, the prevalence of psoriasis is highest in whites (3.6%) followed by blacks (1.9%) and Hispanics (1.6%).[9] The mode of inheritance is intricate and several chromosomal loci are associated with disease.[10] In genetically susceptible individuals, various antigens are capable of activating T cells, resulting in hyperproliferation of keratinocytes, altered epidermal differentiation, and cutaneous inflammation. One antigen in particular, associated with streptococcal infection, has been causally related to onset and flare of psoriasis.[11]

CLINICAL PRESENTATIONS OF PSORIASIS

Five subtypes of psoriasis are recognized: plaque, guttate, pustular, inverse, and erythrodermic.

Plaque psoriasis (**Figs. 1–3**) is the most common presentation, comprising 85% to 90% of all cases.[12] The condition manifests as well-demarcated erythematous plaques with xerotic, silvery scale that can attain several centimeters in diameter. Removal of scales results in punctate bleeding (Auspitz sign). Individual lesions may be irregular, round, or ovoid and may be sparsely located or occur in a generalized distribution covering a majority of the body surface. The most common locations are the scalp, trunk, buttocks, and limbs. Extensor surfaces, such as the elbows and knees, are frequently involved and may be the first and only presentation of disease. Approximately 80% of patients suffer from mild to moderate disease, which covers less than 10% of the body surface area, whereas the remainder are afflicted with moderate to severe disease.[13]

Guttate psoriasis is characterized by 1-mm to 10-mm, pink to erythematous colored papules, often covered with fine scale (**Fig. 4**). This variant of psoriasis most commonly arises in individuals younger than 30 years and is located primarily on the trunk and the proximal extremities, occurring in less than 2% of patients with psoriasis. Guttate psoriasis may be preceded by group A β-hemolytic streptococcal pharyngitis and may improve or resolve with antibiotic therapy or evolve into plaque psoriasis.[14]

Pustular psoriasis is an uncommon subtype that can be divided into generalized and localized forms. The acute generalized form, also known as the von Zumbusch variant, is a severe and explosive condition accompanied by fever that presents with multiple sterile pustules arising on an erythematous or dusky background (**Fig. 5**). Rapid progression and systemic toxicity may be life threatening. Localized forms of pustular

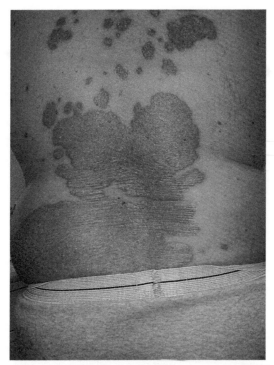

Fig. 1. Well-demarcated erythematous plaques are the hallmark of psoriasis.

psoriasis affect the hands and feet and may be an isolated phenomenon or found in association with plaque psoriasis. Palmoplantar psoriasis is a condition characterized by erythema, fissuring, and scaling. This condition has been linked to cigarette smoking[15] and may improve with cessation.

Inverse psoriasis, also known as flexural or intertriginous psoriasis, is characterized by lesions situated within the skin folds and affects between 3% and 7% of individuals with this disease.[16] Due to the moist and warm nature of these areas, psoriasis localized to folds tends toward erythematous patches with minimal scale (**Fig. 6**). Common sites include the axillary, genital, perineal, and inframammary areas.

Erythrodermic psoriasis (**Fig. 7**) may evolve from chronic plaque disease or develop acutely de novo. It occurs in less than 2% of cases and may involve the entire skin surface.[17] Chills and hypothermia can result from altered thermoregulation and fluid loss may precipitate dehydration. Extensive cases may eventuate in sepsis.

NONDERMATOLOGIC MANIFESTATIONS

Nail disease (psoriatic onychodystrophy) occurs in a majority of persons with psoriasis (**Figs. 8–10**).[18] Fingernails are involved in approximately 50% of all patients and toenails in 35%.[13] Abnormal nail plate growth results in pitting, subungual hyperkeratosis, and the oil-drop sign. Pits are depressions within the nail plate and are the most common nail finding in psoriasis, although not specific for this disease.[19] Subungual hyperkeratosis results from the deposition of cellular debris under the nail plate. Over time

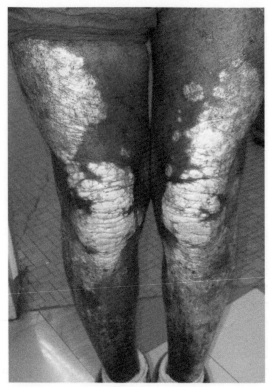

Fig. 2. Plaques of psoriasis manifesting thick adherent scales, which markedly impede penetration of topical therapies.

the nail thickens and becomes more brittle. The primary differential diagnosis is onychomycosis. Oil-drop spots result from psoriatic lesions contained within the nail bed. These are translucent yellowish to pink discolorations that resemble drops of oil under the nail surface.

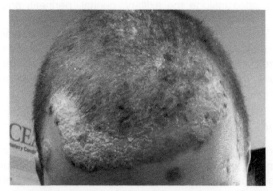

Fig. 3. Scalp psoriasis affects more than 50% of individuals with this disorder. The condition may present with fine scale or, in more severe cases, with thick, crusted plaques that extend onto the forehead and posterior neck.

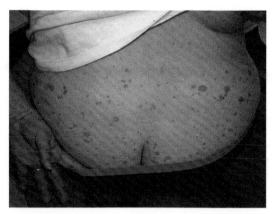

Fig. 4. Guttate psoriasis arises suddenly, concentrates on the trunk, and may be preceded by streptococcal pharyngeal infection.

ARTHRITIS

Psoriatic arthritis (PsA) is a chronic seronegative inflammatory joint arthritis that affects approximately 25% to 30% of individuals with psoriasis.[20] Similar to rheumatoid arthritis, PSA has the potential for joint damage and disability. The condition affects men and women equally and has a peak age of onset of between 35 and 45 years of age. The prevalence increases in individuals with more extensive skin disease. In a majority of patients, skin psoriasis precedes PsA; however, in approximately 15%, the reverse is noted.[21]

PsA may be asymptomatic or associated with pain, tenderness, and swelling of the joints and surrounding ligaments and tendons. The pattern of joint involvement associated with PsA is variable. Unique to PsA is the DIP predominant pattern, which occurs in approximately 10% of patients and primarily in men.[22] Approximately 30% of PsA patients experience asymmetric oligoarticular arthritis with involvement of a large joint, such as the knee, and a few small joints of the hands or feet, often in association with dactylitis. Also common, especially in women, is the polyarthritis

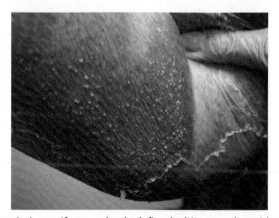

Fig. 5. Pustular psoriasis manifests as clearly defined white pustules arising on an erythematous base. The condition usually arises acutely and be precipitated by medications including lithium and nonsteroidal anti-inflammatory drugs.

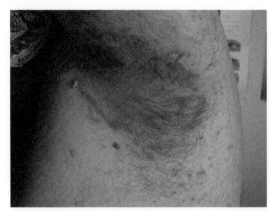

Fig. 6. Inverse psoriasis involves the axillae and intergluteal and crural folds. The male and female genitalia may also be affected. The skin is erythematous and usually devoid of scale.

pattern involving the fingers, wrists, toes, and ankles in a symmetric distribution. The most debilitating form of PsA is called arthritis mutilans, characterized by bone absorption and deformity.

Associated with PsA may be enthesitis, or inflammation at the site of tendon or ligament insertion into bone. Common sites include the insertion zones of the plantar fascia, the Achilles tendons, and ligament attachments to the ribs, spine, and pelvis.

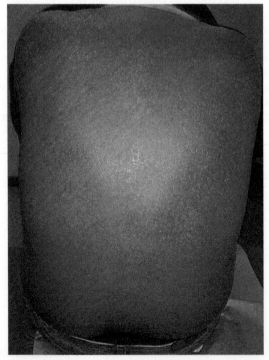

Fig. 7. Erythrodermic psoriasis is an uncommon variant that covers much of the body surface, including the face and hands. Patients may present with fever, chills, and dehydration.

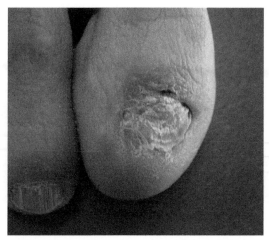

Fig. 8. Nail deformity secondary to psoriasis. Nail psoriasis is a common manifestation of this disease and may present with onycholysis, pitting, and discoloration.

Dactylitis, or sausage digit, is a combination of enthesitis of the tendons and ligaments accompanied by synovitis involving a whole digit. The toes are most commonly affected.[23]

COMORBIDITIES

Several prospective and retrospective studies have validated the association of psoriasis and PsA with diabetes, hyperlipidemia, hypertension, atherosclerosis, and myocardial infection.[24–28] The chronic inflammatory response that underlies psoriasis is believed to play a key role in the pathogenesis of these adverse events as well. Because such conditions adversely affect morbidity and mortality in patients with psoriasis, comprehensive management best includes screening, monitoring, and,

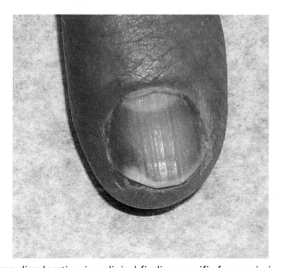

Fig. 9. The oil drop discoloration is a clinical finding specific for psoriasis.

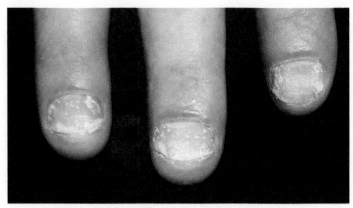

Fig. 10. Pitting of nails frequently accompanies psoriasis and most commonly affects the fingernails.

when indicated, prompt intervention. Treatment strategies for controlling moderate to severe disease may have a favorable impact on cardiovascular endpoints.

TREATMENT

Treatment goals are control and improvement of disease and symptoms. More recently, dampening of the chronic inflammatory response has been advocated to decrease overall morbidity and mortality. A survey by the National Psoriasis Foundation revealed that a significant proportion of individuals with moderate to severe psoriasis receive no treatment or are undertreated.[29] Factors for this disparity include the high cost of medications and difficulty accessing medical specialists experienced in disease management, namely dermatologists and rheumatologists.

Topical Therapies

Topical therapies are a mainstay in the management of mild disease.[30] Disadvantages include the time required for application, local adverse reactions, and incomplete lesion clearance.

Topical corticosteroids are considered first-line therapy for less extensive disease due to their anti-inflammatory properties. Initial treatment often entails use of superpotent formulations, which are available as creams, ointments, gels, lotions, and foams. Examples include clobetasone, betamethasone, and halobetasol. Use for extended periods of time, on the face, axillae, and crural areas or under occlusion, may induce atrophy, telangiectasias, and striae. Midpotency topical steroids, such as triamcinolone, mometasone, and fluticasone, are commonly used as maintenance therapy. The least potent topical steroid, hydrocortisone, is available without prescription (up to 1%) and is safe to use for extended periods on the face and body folds.

Vitamin D analogs, calcipotriene, calcipotriol, and calcitriol, are other first-line topical agents with proved efficacy in the treatment of psoriasis. Calcipotriene/betamethasone diproprionate combines a vitamin D analog with a high-potency topical steroid for enhanced efficacy. Vitamin D analogs affect cellular differentiation and proliferation.

Tazarotene is a vitamin A derivative approved to treat psoriasis. This medication diminishes epidermal turnover and inflammation. Erythema, burning, and pruritus may limit use and the drug is contraindicated during pregnancy.

Phototherapy

Cabinet-based UV light therapy has been used for decades to treat widespread psoriasis or disease that is refractory to topical therapies. Wavelength in the narrow-band–UV-B spectrum is the preferred phototherapy modality and is safe to use in both children and pregnant women.[31] Treatment is ideally performed 3 times per week over a several-month period. Home-based units are available and effective. The efficacy of narrowband–UV-B may be enhanced in combination with other treatment modalities.

Oral systemic therapies

Acitretin (Soriatane) is an oral retinoid with daily dosing that ranges from 10 mg to 50 mg. Retinoids modulate epidermal proliferation and differentiation and exhibit anti-inflammatory properties. The drug is teratogenic and must not be taken by pregnant women or those contemplating pregnancy within a 3-year time frame. Skin and lip dryness and hair loss are the most common adverse events. The drug can elevate serum triglycerides, necessitating periodic laboratory monitoring.

Apremilast (Otezla) is a phosphodiesterase type 4 inhibitor approved in 2014 for the treatment of moderate to severe psoriasis and PsA. The medication is taken twice daily, at a dose of 30 mg. In clinical studies, a response equal to or greater than 75% was achieved in 29% to 33% of patients. Routine laboratory studies are not required. The most common adverse events are diarrhea and nausea, which tend to dissipate with continued therapy.

Cyclosporine (Neoral) is a calcineurin inhibitor that dampens T-cell activation. The drug is administered on a daily basis, in a dosing range of 2.5 mg/kg to 5 mg/kg; works rapidly; and has the highest efficacy of all systemic therapies. Cyclosporine may raise serum triglycerides and blood pressure. Long-term use may cause renal impairment and periodic laboratory monitoring is mandatory.

Methotrexate has been used to treat psoriasis for more than 50 years. The drug inhibits epidermal cell division and is usually administered on a once-weekly basis with dosage varying between 5 mg/wk and 25 mg/wk. The drug is immunosuppressive and should not be used in patients with active infections. It is contraindicated in pregnancy but safe to use in pediatric patients. Hepatotoxicity is the most common serious adverse event and is most likely to occur in persons who are obese or diabetic.

Biologics

Biologic agents are protein-based compounds made from living cells that mitigate against inflammatory agents involved in the pathogenesis of psoriatic plaques and arthritis. These medications allow physicians to directly target mediators of the immune system that induce psoriasis and have revolutionized therapy for this disease. Currently approved biologic agents for the treatment of psoriasis include the following:

- TNF inhibitors: adalimumab (Humira), etanercept (Enbrel), and infliximab (Remicade)
- IL-12/23 inhibitors: ustekinumab (Stelara)
- IL-17 inhibitor: secukinumab (Cosentyx)

Adalimumab

Adalimumab is a recombinant IgG1 antibody that binds specifically to TNF-α and blocks its interaction with key cell surface TNF receptors. The drug was approved to treat psoriasis in 2008. For psoriasis, an initial dose of 80 mg is given subcutaneously followed 1 week later by 40 mg, with this dose then continued every other week.

Etanercept

Etanercept is a fusion protein approved in 2004 for the treatment of psoriasis. It inhibits binding of TNF-α and TNF-β to cell surface TNF receptors. The drug is administered by subcutaneous injection. For psoriasis, the starting dose is 50 mg twice weekly for 3 months, followed by 50 mg weekly.

Infliximab

Infliximab is a chimeric IgG1κ monoclonal antibody specific for human TNF-α approved to treat psoriasis in 2006. The drug neutralizes TNF-α by inhibiting binding to receptor sites. For plaque psoriasis, the recommended dose is 5 mg/kg given as an intravenous induction regimen at 0, 2, and 6 weeks followed by a maintenance regimen of 5 mg/kg every 8 weeks thereafter.

Ustekinumab

Ustekinumab is a human IgG1κ monoclonal antibody that binds to the p40 protein subunit used by both IL-12 and IL-23 cytokines. Approved in 2009 to treat psoriasis, the drug is administered subcutaneously with dosage dependent on weight. For patients under 100 kg, the recommended dose is 45 mg initially and 4 weeks later, followed by 45 mg every 12 weeks. Heavier individuals are treated with 90 mg at the same dosing schedule.

Secukinumab

Secukinumab was approved to treat psoriasis in January 2015. The drug is a human IgG1κ monoclonal antibody that binds and inhibits IL-17A. The recommended dose is 300 mg by subcutaneous injection at weeks 0, 1, 2, 3, and 4 followed by 300 mg every 4 weeks.

Concerns have been raised about potential long-term sequelae associated with systemic and biologic psoriasis therapies[32]; fortunately, the safety track record to date is favorable regarding incidence of serious infections, major cardiac events, and malignancies.[33] When using immune-modulating agents, initial screening should include assays for hepatitis B, hepatitis C, and tuberculosis, with testing for tuberculosis exposure repeated on a yearly basis.

Psoriasis is a complex disorder that involves genetic, environmental, and immunologic factors.[34] The disorder has no known cure but today an overwhelming majority of patients can achieve good to excellent control. A multitude of promising therapies are in the pipeline,[35-37] some nearing Food and Drug Administration approval. There are significant barriers to optimal management, which include expense, patient compliance, and medication safety. When dealing with this disease, health care providers should strive to identify the most efficacious treatment associated with the fewest possible adverse events delivered at a reasonable cost.

Podiatrists may encounter several variants of psoriasis, including the palmarplantar subtype, nail disease, and arthritis. Palmar-plantar psoriasis may be debilitating and is often refractory to topical therapies (ultrapotent topical steroids, retinoids, and calcipotriol) necessitating phototherapy, oral systemics (ie, acitretin or methotrexate), or biologics. Painful or disfiguring nail distortion may respond to intralesional steroid injections administered to the nail base as well as to systemic or biologic therapy. A multidisciplinary approach to achieve ideal control is highly recommended and should include a dermatologist, for management of moderate to severe skin and nail disease, and a rheumatologist, for management of joint disease. Given the significant comorbidities associated with psoriasis, such as diabetes, hypertension, and hyperlipidemia, consultation with other specialists may be prudent as well.

REFERENCES

1. Kurd SK, Gelfand JM. The prevalence of previously diagnosed and undiagnosed psoriasis in US adults: results from NHANES 2003-2004. J Am Acad Dermatol 2009;60(2):218–24.
2. Christophers E. Psoriasis–epidemiology and clinical spectrum. Clin Exp Dermatol 2001;26(4):314–20.
3. Raychaudhuri SP, Farber EM. The prevalence of psoriasis in the world. J Eur Acad Dermatol Venereol 2001;15(1):16–7.
4. Kimball AB, Jacobson C, Weiss S, et al. The psychosocial burden of psoriasis. Am J Clin Dermatol 2005;6(6):383–92.
5. Armstrong AW, Schupp C, Wu J, et al. Quality of life and work productivity impairment among psoriasis patients: findings from the National Psoriasis Foundation survey data 2003-2011. PLoS One 2012;7(12):e52935.
6. Brezinski EA, Dhillon JS, Armstrong AW. Economic burden of psoriasis in the United States: a systematic review. JAMA Dermatol 2015;151(6):651–8.
7. Sabat R, Philipp S, Höflich C, et al. Immunopathogenesis of psoriasis. Exp Dermatol 2007;16(10):779–98.
8. Farber EM, Nall ML. The natural history of psoriasis in 5,600 patients. Dermatologica 1974;148:1–18.
9. Rachakonda TD, Schupp CW, Armstrong AW. Psoriasis prevalence among adults in the United States. J Am Acad Dermatol 2014;70(3):512–6.
10. Cargill M, Schrodi SJ, Chang M, et al. A large-scale genetic association study confirms IL12B and leads to the identification of IL23R as psoriasis-risk genes. Am J Hum Genet 2007;80(2):273–90.
11. Telfer NR, Chalmers RJ, Whale K, et al. The role of streptococcal infection in the initiation of guttate psoriasis. Arch Dermatol 1992;128:39–42.
12. Nestle FO, Kaplan DH, Barker J. Psoriasis. N Engl J Med 2009;361(5):496–509.
13. Menter A, Gottlieb A, Feldman SR, et al. Guidelines of care for the management of psoriasis and psoriatic arthritis: section 1. Overview of psoriasis and guidelines of care for the treatment of psoriasis with biologics. J Am Acad Dermatol 2008; 58(5):826–50.
14. Martin BA, Chalmers RJ, Telfer NR. How great is the risk of further psoriasis following a single episode of acute guttate psoriasis? Arch Dermatol 1996; 132(6):717–8.
15. Naldi L, Chatenoud L, Linder D, et al. Cigarette smoking, body mass index, and stressful life events as risk factors for psoriasis: results from an Italian case-control study. J Invest Dermatol 2005;125(1):61–7.
16. Guglielmetti A, Conlledo R, Bedoya J, et al. Inverse psoriasis involving genital skin folds. Dermatol Ther (Heidelb) 2012;2(1):1.
17. Lebwohl M. Psoriasis. Lancet 2003;361:1197–204.
18. Reich K. Approach to managing patients with nail psoriasis. J Eur Acad Dermatol Venereol 2009;23(Suppl 1):15–21.
19. Jiaravuthisan MM, Sasseville D, Vender RB, et al. Psoriasis of the nail: anatomy, pathology, clinical presentation, and a review of the literature on therapy. J Am Acad Dermatol 2007;57(1):1–27.
20. Menter A, Korman NJ, Elmets CA, et al. Guidelines of care for the management of psoriasis and psoriatic arthritis: section 6. Guidelines of care for the treatment of psoriasis and psoriatic arthritis: case-based presentations and evidence-based conclusions. J Am Acad Dermatol 2011;65(1):137–74.

21. Gladman DD, Shuckett R, Russell ML, et al. Psoriatic arthritis (PSA)—an analysis of 220 patients. Q J Med 1987;62:127–41.
22. Khan M, Schentag C, Gladman DD. Clinical and radiological changes during psoriatic arthritis disease progression. J Rheumatol 2003;30:1022–6.
23. Brockbank JE, Stein M, Schentag CT, et al. Dactylitis in psoriatic arthritis: a marker for disease severity. Ann Rheum Dis 2005;64:188–90.
24. Mehta NN, Azfar RS, Shin DB, et al. Patients with severe psoriasis are at increased risk of cardiovascular mortality: cohort study using the general practice research database. Eur Heart J 2010;31(8):1000–6.
25. Gelfand JM, Neimann AL, Shin DB, et al. Risk of myocardial infarction in patients with psoriasis. JAMA 2006;296(14):1735–41.
26. Shlyankevich J, Mehta NN, Krueger JG, et al. Accumulating evidence for the association and shared pathogenic mechanisms between psoriasis and cardiovascular-related comorbidities. Am J Med 2014;127(12):1148–53.
27. Cohen AD, Dreiher J, Shapiro Y, et al. Psoriasis and diabetes: a population-based cross-sectional study. J Eur Acad Dermatol Venereol 2008;22(5):585–9.
28. Horreau C, Pouplard C, Brenaut E, et al. Cardiovascular morbidity and mortality in psoriasis and psoriatic arthritis: a systematic literature review. J Eur Acad Dermatol Venereol 2013;27(Suppl 3):12–29.
29. Armstrong AW, Robertson AD, Wu J, et al. Undertreatment, treatment trends, and treatment dissatisfaction among patients with psoriasis and psoriatic arthritis in the United States: findings from the National Psoriasis Foundation surveys, 2003-2011. JAMA Dermatol 2013;149(10):1180–5.
30. Menter A, Korman NJ, Elmets CA, et al. Guidelines of care for the management of psoriasis and psoriatic arthritis. Section 3. Guidelines of care for the management and treatment of psoriasis with topical therapies. J Am Acad Dermatol 2009; 60(4):643–59.
31. Lapolla W, Yentzer BA, Bagel J, et al. A review of phototherapy protocols for psoriasis treatment. J Am Acad Dermatol 2011;64(5):936–49.
32. Schleicher SM. Efficacy and emergent sequelae in the use of biologics for psoriasis. Emerg Med 2010;42(4):6–11.
33. Reich K, Mrowietz U. Drug safety of systemic treatments for psoriasis: results from The German Psoriasis Registry PsoBest. Arch Dermatol Res 2015; 307(10):875–83.
34. Ryan C, Korman NJ, Gelfand JM, et al. Research gaps in psoriasis: opportunities for future studies. J Am Acad Dermatol 2014;70(1):146–67.
35. Feely MA, Smith BL, Weinberg JM. Novel psoriasis therapies and patient outcomes, part 1: topical medications. Cutis 2015;95(3):164–8.
36. Feely MA, Smith BL, Weinberg JM. Novel psoriasis therapies and patient outcomes, part 2: biologic treatments. Cutis 2015;95(5):282–90.
37. Feely MA, Smith BL, Weinberg JM. Novel psoriasis therapies and patient outcomes, Part 3: systemic medications. Cutis 2015;96(1):47–53.

Dermatologic Concerns of the Lower Extremity in the Pediatric Patient

Tracey C. Vlahovic, DPM, FFPM RCPS (Glasg)

KEYWORDS

- Pediatrics • Warts • Genodermatoses • Sweaty sock dermatitis • Psoriasis
- Eczema

KEY POINTS

- Cutaneous disorders of the lower extremity in pediatric patients deserve special attention because their body surface area differs from that in adult patients.
- Special care should be taken in educating parents and making children comfortable if a procedure is necessary on the lower extremity.
- Various skin conditions, ranging from environmental to infectious, can be seen and treated on the lower extremity in pediatric patients.

DIAGNOSING SKIN DISEASE IN THE PEDIATRIC POPULATION

A pediatric patient presenting with a skin condition can prove a challenge to diagnose and manage. When faced with a patient with a skin condition in the office, the practitioner should have a systematic approach to arrive at a baseline differential diagnosis: observe and ask. After clinically visualizing the lesion, it may be helpful to perform a skin biopsy to refine the diagnosis or, in some cases, act as a therapeutic tool to excise the lesion.

Observe

On entering a treatment room, the practitioner should notice the color, shape, and size in addition to laterality of the patient's lesions on the lower extremity.[1] Primary and secondary lesions (macules, pustules, vesicles, and so forth) should be used to describe the rash appropriately both in the chart and in correspondence to other physicians. When looking at the shape of the lesions, it is helpful to determine if they are self-induced by the patient (excoriation by a fingernail) or naturally caused (scaly skin). The practitioner should document if the lesions are plantar foot, dorsal foot, or headed proximally on the lower leg. Nail involvement should be noted. Finally, the fingernails

Department of Podiatric Medicine, Temple University School of Podiatric Medicine, 148 North 8th Street, Philadelphia, PA 19107, USA
E-mail address: traceyv@temple.edu

Clin Podiatr Med Surg 33 (2016) 367–384
http://dx.doi.org/10.1016/j.cpm.2016.02.005
0891-8422/16/$ – see front matter © 2016 Elsevier Inc. All rights reserved.

and dorsum and palmar aspects of the hands should be examined because many skin dermatoses mirror the pedal involvement there.

Ask

Questions that help form differential diagnoses should be asked when completing the physical examination of the skin. Often, a patient answers a question that helps direct the diagnosis, but in pediatric patients, interview of the guardian is paramount. Beyond asking the history of present illness, past medical history, and family history, the physician should consider asking if there is a personal or family history of allergic rhinitis, sensitive skin, asthma, or skin cancer. Patients should be asked if they had ever seen a specialist before and if they have any skin lesions (or rashes) anywhere else on the body that may or may not be similar to what is seen on the lower extremity. Unfortunately, most patients do not correlate what is happening on the rest of the body to what is manifesting on the plantar aspect of the feet. It is the physician's responsibility to ask the questions to make that connection. It is helpful to ask if the skin has ever been biopsied (for example, "Did you have a piece of skin removed and then have stitches?"). A skin scraping for potassium hydroxide (KOH) that was completed by another physician does not count as a proper biopsy to base a diagnosis on, because a biopsy of inflammatory skin disorders should include the dermis from a pathology perspective. Other questions to consider asking patients are the color of socks they wear (azo dyes in blue socks can be a potential allergen), daily recreational activities, and any associated daily hazards. Also, they should be asked about both over-the-counter and homeopathic or natural treatment options they have tried. To plan for a possible in-office biopsy that visit, it is important to ask what the natural progression of the lesions has been and where the newest crop of lesions are.

After the basic observation and questioning have occurred, it is important to delve more deeply into the chief complaint and examine the skin fully.

A Note on Skin Biopsies and Other Cutaneous Procedures in the Pediatric Patient

Many of the following skin issues discussed in this article may require a skin biopsy as a diagnostic and therapeutic tool. It is important to consider the following when performing a cutaneous procedure.

First, consider the parent. After explaining thoroughly the procedure to the parent, the practitioner may give the parent a job to assist during the procedure. This may consist of the parent holding the child in his or her lap or distracting the child during the injection.

Second, making the child comfortable before, during, and after the procedure is paramount. For example, application of topical lidocaine to the area in question may be helpful in easing pain from the initial needle stick.[2] Also, pinching, rubbing, or vibration of the skin prior to injection may reduce pain from the injection. During the injection process itself, techniques of distraction, such as blowing soap bubbles, allowing the child to hold a favorite toy, listening to music with headphones, and conversing with the child, can be used.[3] These methods, followed by positive feedback verbally or with an object (a toy or sticker), reduce the overall anxiety caused by the procedure.

Dealing with an older child requires discussing the procedure in simple terms directly to the patient and describing how the injection or procedure will feel. Again, during and after the procedure, conversing with and rewarding the patient may make the overall experience a comfortable one for the child.

Lastly, it is important to set limits for the child postoperatively to have the best scar outcome. This is particularly relevant for the plantar foot. The use of crutches and off-loading techniques coupled with a decrease of gym and sports activity may be necessary to recommend during the postoperative recovery period.

ENVIRONMENTALLY INDUCED SKIN DISORDERS

When the skin barrier is compromised from the weather, insects, or trauma, the skin reacts in various ways.

Sun Exposure

Sunburn is an inflammatory reaction to the cellular damage from UV-B radiation.[4] It presents as pain and tenderness of the skin with an erythematous discoloration progressing to desquamation. More severe cases are accompanied by fatigue, headache, and chills. Treatment consists of local support—topical corticosteroids, cooling baths, emollient creams, oral nonsteroidal anti-inflammatory medications, and hydration.

The depth of a tan, whether from a tanning salon bed or environmental exposure, is a direct correlation of the amount of UV radiation absorbed by the skin. Because radiation damages the cells, melanocytes are activated and produce more melanosomes. The melanosomes, or sacs containing pigment, are then transferred to the keratinocytes.[4] Long-term sequelae of tanning include photodamage (wrinkles and pigmentation) and a decreased immune response of the processes suppressing conditions, like herpes simplex virus and nonmelanoma skin cancer.

Heat and Cold

Burns from heat may be caused by dry or wet heat as well as chemicals. They are classified on the depth of damage involved within the epidermis and dermis. Children are more prone to scalding burns from touching hot drinks or bath water. Localized bullae after the injury may be treated with local wound care, but more extensive and deeper burns require admission to a facility for intravenous fluid replacement, débridement of devitalized tissue, analgesics, antibiotics, and possible skin grafting or amputation depending on the extent of injury.

Pernio is a nonfreezing injury that occurs in response to repeated cold exposure with humid conditions and manifests itself as erythematous to violaceous papules, nodules, or plaques that may burn, be pruritic, or become vesicles. This typically happens on toes and fingers. The lesions may occur 24 hours after exposure and last from 1 to 3 weeks. Warming the affected part and wearing appropriate clothing during future cold exposure are helpful in treatment and prevention.

Frostnip is a milder form of cold injury compared with pernio. It generally occurs on the most distal aspects: toes, fingers, nose, and ears. It represents a superficial injury to the skin and manifests itself as blanching of the skin and numbness.[5] It is reversible on rewarming of the part and preventing further cold exposure.

Due to the similarity of the injury to burns, frostbite is classified as first-degree, second-degree, third-degree, and fourth-degree injuries; however, most physicians classify it either as superficial (first-degree and second-degree) or deep (third-degree and fourth-degree). On initial presentation, it is difficult to tell which degree of frostbite is present.[6] Only after rewarming can a clinician tell how deeply the layers of the skin and subcutaneous tissue have been affected. The skin and subcutaneous tissue are affected in superficial frostbite, which may manifest as nonblanching anesthetic white waxy skin, which becomes painful on thawing as well as edematous with serous vesicles and bullae. Deep frostbite goes beyond the skin and subcutaneous tissues into the muscles, neurovascular structures, and bone. The frozen part may look wooden and have a lack of sensation that may look ashen on rewarming.[7] Hemorrhagic bullae may form eventually.

After removing the patient from the environment, rapid rewarming in a bath of 39°C to 42°C is indicated. Tetanus status should be verified because these injuries can be tetanus-prone.

Bites and Stings and Infestations

Having an insect sting or bite is a common occurrence of childhood. First, it is important to distinguish between bites and stings. An insect bite from the mouth parts is to feed from the host whereas a sting is in self-defense. Most of the time, an insect (in particular, a bee) can sting only once but can bite multiple times. In certain cases, an insect, such as the wasp, can both sting and bite at the same time. In podiatric medicine, a child playing or running without shoes makes the lower extremity particularly vulnerable to the following issues.

Hymenoptera include bees, wasps, and ants whose stings can cause both local and systemic (anaphylaxis) reactions. Local reactions may appear as an urticarial wheal with a central puncture mark that may in time become excoriated by the patient. A mild reaction may be treated with ice and an oral antihistamine whereas a more severe local reaction requires systemic corticosteroids.[8] Anaphylaxis should be treated with a subcutaneous or intramuscular injection of epinephrine (0.01 mg/kg) and the emergency response system should be activated. If not treated, anaphylaxis may lead to death. In addition, a high number of stings (500–1000) may also lead to death.

Scabies is from the human scabies mite known as *Sarcoptes scabiei* var. *hominis*. The mode of transmission is usually from an infected person in close contact with the patient but the mite can also live several days on fomites, such as bed linen.[9] A hallmark of the infestation is an intractable itch that is worse at night. The pathognomonic lesion is a burrow which may present as a small grayish line at the interdigital webs of the hands and feet, anterior wrists, axillary folds, and ankles. In young children, an extensive eczematous eruption on the trunk or chest may appear.[10] Infants may have papules and vesicles on the palms and soles.[10] The intense pruritus associated with these lesions converts the burrows into excoriations and possibly secondarily infected lesions.

A skin scraping of the infested site may confirm the presence of the mite as well as its larvae, ova, and fecal matter. As soon as a diagnosis is made, the patient, all of the contacts, bed linens, and clothing should be treated or laundered. Permethrin 5% is the topical treatment of choice in infants and small children and is applied from head to toe once weekly for a minimum of 2 consecutive weeks.

Trauma

Burns from electrical wires and lightning can occur in the pediatric population. Electrical wire injuries are seen in children 6 and younger and lightning injuries can occur in a child who enjoys the outdoors.[4] Treatment can range from supportive to resuscitative depending on the severity. With the local supportive care, it is important for tetanus prophylaxis to be up to date.

Both human-caused and animal-caused bites can be a source of trauma to the pediatric patient. Human bites may come from aggressive play with another child and can present as superficial semicircular contusions, scratches, or lacerations.[11] They more commonly occur on the upper extremity but can occur on the lower extremity. Infection is the most common complication and local wound care should be initiated as soon as possible.

A child wearing new, ill-fitting shoes may cause vesicles or bullae to form, especially in the presence of hyperhidrosis. These lesions may or may not be drained, but local wound care and protection of the lesions should be considered.

Talon noir, or calcaneal petechiae, is a nonpainful, self-limiting lesion that can arise after sports in young adults.[12] It is a result of continuous lateral shearing force in the shoe. It has been classically described after playing basketball but can occur in any sport that has frequent stops and starts. The small macules are located over the posterior to posterolateral aspect of the calcaneus and resolve on their own.

Unusual and repeated patterns of bruising, such as those caused by an electrical cord, knuckles, or another instrument, and bullae from burns may be seen in child abuse cases.[13] Child abuse should be considered a differential diagnosis in these cases but also should be diagnosed with certainty. It is imperative to diagnose this correctly because missing it can have tragic consequences for the child.

GENODERMATOSES

Genodermatoses, or inherited skin conditions, contain a subset of hereditary palmoplantar keratodermas (PPKs). These genetic skin disorders characteristically involve hyperkeratosis of the palms and soles.[14] The patterns of hyperkeratosis are further divided into diffuse and focal groups.

Vörner-Unna-Thost Type

Also known as epidermolytic palmoplantar hyperkeratosis or Unna-Thost type, the Vörner-Unna-Thost PPK type is the most common of these genetically based hyperkeratotic disorders a practitioner encounters, at a rate of 1:100,000. It is inherited autosomally dominantly with mutations seen in keratins 9 and 1. It clinically presents as diffuse areas of yellow hyperkeratotic plaques on the palms and soles surrounded by an erythematous border. Nail changes and fungal superinfections also may be seen.

Vohwinkel Type

The Vohwinkel PPK type is also known as keratosis palmoplantaris mutilans and mutilating keratoderma with deafness. It is a dominant-negative mutation for the genes that code for connexin 26. This ultimately can affect both hearing and skin. The plantar and palmar skin appears as diffuse honeycombed yellow hyperkeratosis with hyperhidrosis. Over time, constrictions can occur at the distal joints, which may lead to pseudoainhum and, ultimately, autoamputation.

Pachyonychia Congenita

There are 2 types of pachyonychia congenita: type I (Jadassohn-Lewandowsky type) and type II (Jackson-Lawler type). It is also inherited in an autosomal-dominant fashion with mutations in keratin 6a and keratin 16 in type I and mutations in keratin 6b and keratin 17 in type II. In this type of PPK, the main skin appendage affected is the nails. Nails, shortly after birth, become hyperkeratotic and dystrophic. Focal plantar hyperkertoses over pressure points may also develop.

Tuberous Sclerosis

Although not a PPK, tuberous sclerosis is inherited by autosomal dominance. This disease is often associated with multiple periungual fibromas around the nail unit, which makes nail débridement challenging. These numerous fibromas, or Koenen tumors, may distort the nail plate. Also associated with tuberous sclerosis are areas of hypopigmentation, which, when illuminated with a Wood lamp, appear as ash tree leaves.

Treatment of Genodermatoses

There is a lack of randomized controlled studies due to the small size of this patient population. First-line therapy generally consists of a topical keratolytic to aid in desquamation. Choices include urea (10%–40%), salicylic acid (6%), and lactic acid (12%). Physicians should also consider the prophylactic use of topical antifungal therapies that can occur in patients with concurrent hyperhidrosis.[14] Further therapies beyond topical medications are skin and nail débridement by a physician, soaking and use of pumice stone by the patient, laser ablation, and lastly surgical débridement followed by a skin graft.[15] The systemic retinoid acitretin is used long term to decrease many side effects, but, as always, benefit should outweigh risk because the side effects of retinoids should be considered (premature growth plate closure, elevated serum fats, and osteoporosis).[14] Genetic counseling should be considered in this patient population.

BACTERIAL INFECTIONS

Bacterial infections can generally be divided into staphylococcus-caused and streptococcus-caused infections. Community-acquired methicillin-resistant *Staphylococcus aureus* is widely prevalent and should now be ruled out as a pathogen for simple lesions, such as carbuncles and paronychias of the great toe. Corynebacterium and pseudomonas can also be pathogens. The type of bacteria and the level of skin invasion present with characteristic skin conditions. If the infection is severe and not treated, complications, such as sepsis, kidney failure, and heart disease, may occur.[16]

Impetigo

Staphylococci or group A streptococcus pyogenes may penetrate a skin abrasion and cause blistering. If it is staphylococcus induced, the blister may be a flaccid blister with lakes of purulence visible. If caused by streptococcus, the blister is fragile and on breaking forms a honey-colored crustlike appearance. It is extremely contagious. For a localized skin reaction of either the bullous or nonbullous type, topical mupirocin or retapamulin may be applied. For a more extensive presentation, oral dicloxacillin or cefazolin may be prescribed for 7 to 10 days.[17]

Cellulitis

Cellulitis may also be caused by staphylococcus or streptococcus and penetrates through a wound or a macerated area. First presentation may be a localized area of erythema, calor, edema, or dolor that may progress to lymphangitis or erythematous streaking proximally; lymphadenopathy; and constitutional signs and symptoms (fever, malaise, and chills). Treatment is generally application of intravenous antibiotics, such as a combination of cefazolin/clindamycin or linezolid alone in addition to an incision and drainage of a distal abscess, if present.[17]

Folliculitis

Inflammation and colonization of the hair follicles may present with tender, irritated areas. Folliculits may start out as a pustule or erythematous papule around the hair unit and may progress to the staphylococcus-induced furuncle (boil) and ultimately a network of furuncles or a carbuncle. The treatment of carbuncles generally involves incision and drainage as well as systemic antibiotic therapy. Folliculitis may also be caused by a dermatophyte and pseudomonas, and systemic therapies should be targeted for those organisms.

Pitted Keratolysis/Erythrasma

A superficial infection of the intertriginous areas of the skin, such as the interdigital web spaces by *Corynebacterium minutissimum*, produces erythrasma. Erythrasma may appear as a macerated interdigital infection with some scale and malodor. On illumination under a Wood lamp, corynebacterium fluoresces coral red or, if caused by pseudomonas, fluoresces green. Pitted keratolysis is a superficial infection also caused mainly by corynebacterium on the plantar aspect of the foot. It is characterized by tiny craters and maceration. It generally does not fluoresce under a Wood lamp. Classically, this is treated with a topical antibiotic, such as clindamycin or erythromycin, and a drying agent, like aluminum chloride solution.

Pseudomonas Hot Foot Syndrome

Pseudomonal infections of the nail and skin commonly occur after immersion in water colonized with the gram-negative rod. Pseudomonas hot foot syndrome describes tender, erythematous nodules on the plantar aspect of the feet that develop after swimming in colonized pool water. It is a benign, self-limiting disease that may or may not require systemic antibiotics depending on the case.[18]

VIRAL INFECTIONS
Viral Exanthems

Exanthems are skin manifestations, presenting either directly by a viral infection or indirectly by a child's immune response. They generally occur quickly and can occur on multiple anatomic sites at the same time.[19]

Measles

Measles causes a direct or infectious exanthem by a single-stranded RNA virus belonging to the genus *Morbillivirus*. After transmission from respiratory droplets of an infected individual, an incubation period of 8 to 10 days yields a prodrome of fever, runny nose, cough that worsens at night, conjunctivitis, and Koplik spots, which are pathognomonic grains of salt–appearing dots on the red buccal mucosa. After a few days, the exanthem starts around the ears and then spreads to the rest of the body. It is a maculopapular rash that begins to desquamate in 4 to 7 days after its initial presentation. On the hands and feet, marked desquamation may occur.

Rubella

An RNA virus, rubella is also spread by respiratory droplets. After a prodrome, a cervical lymphadenopathy and a macular facial rash occur and then proceed to work their way distally. The exanthema may disappear in 1 to 3 days, and the signs and symptoms may not occur in 50% of the individuals infected. Diagnosis is key in pregnant women to prevent the complications of rubella (ie, spontaneous abortion or deformity of the fetus).

Fifth disease or erythema infectiosum

Parvovirus B19 is a DNA virus that on transmission via respiratory droplets may cause a slapped cheek appearance in a child 1 to 2 weeks after infection. A reticular or red lacy pattern may occur on the arms, trunk, and legs. This exanthem may fade and reappear after hot baths or exposure to warm temperatures. On the hands and feet, it may appear as a papular rash in a sock-and-glove distribution.

Varicella Zoster

Human herpesvirus type 3 (HHV-3), also known as the varicella zoster virus, is the cause for varicella, commonly known as chickenpox. It is an example of a nondirect viral exanthem. It is highly contagious; therefore, a child with skin disease can transmit the virus as long as there are open lesions present. After an incubation period of 2 weeks, a prodrome occurs and a maculopapular rash begins at the hairline and moves distally, involving both skin and mucous membranes. Its lifespan runs from macule to papule to tense vesicle, followed by pustule, crust, and scar. It is intensely pruritic and may leave a scar. Lesions at different stages appearing simultaneously may be seen on the trunk. It may also affect the hands and feet, including the interdigital areas.[20]

Herpes zoster, or shingles, is the reactivation of HHV-3 that is latent in the dorsal root ganglia. During times of reduced immunity, sunburn, and infection, the virus may awake from its latent state and pass down the nerve to form crops of blisters on a red base. It generally occurs in a unilateral dermatome, but on the lower extremity, it may overlap several dermatomes.

Herpes simplex
The DNA herpes simplex virus (herpes simplex virus 1 and herpes simplex virus 2) also remains in the dorsal root ganglia after an illness. It is reactivated by illness, sunburn, and various triggers and presents as a crop of vesicles on a red base. It is also preceded by a painful stinging sensation. Commonly seen on the face, it may occur on the lower extremity on a digit, termed *herpetic whitlow*.

Hand-foot-and-mouth disease
Hand-foot-and-mouth disease is generally caused by the coxsackievirus A16 enterovirus, which is transmitted by coming into close contact with a young patient. It is highly contagious. After a prodrome of a sore throat and malaise, gray oval-shaped vesicles surrounded by an erythematous halo present on the lateral and medial aspects of the digits in addition to the palmoplantar surfaces. Painful blisters may occur in the mouth. The lesions are self-limiting and typically disappear within 1 week.

Molluscum Contagiosum
Molluscum contagiosum is extremely common in children, where it presents as a flesh-colored, dome-shaped papule that is umbilicated in the center. It is caused by a poxvirus and may resolve on its own in 6 months to a year. It is often found near the axillae and groin. Multiple therapies have been used to treat the lesions (ie, cryotherapy, cantharidin application, and curettage).[21] It may occur extensively in patients with atopic eczema and immunosuppression or in scattered clusters on various sites of the body.

Verrucae
Human papilloma virus (HPV), a DNA virus, is responsible for verrucae, or plantar warts. On the hands and feet, the HPV subtypes are typically 1, 2, and 4. The virus needs an epidermal abrasion and a transiently impaired immune system to inoculate keratinocyte. Showers and swimming pools with abrasive nonslip surfaces act as high-risk areas for simultaneously harboring the virus and causing an epidermal abrasion; 30% of warts may clear spontaneously, but those that do not often are cosmetically unappealing, painful, and irritating to patients. The virus seems to encourage basal cell replication. Hyperplasia of the granular and prickle cell layer occurs, in addition to the dermal papillae arching its vasculature up into the wart. Keratinocytes, with an eccentric nuclei surrounded by a halo (koilocytes), show viral damage of the cells.

Plantar warts are clinically defined as well-circumscribed lesions with overlying hyperkeratosis. On débridement of the hyperkeratosis, pinpoint bleeding and interruption of the skin lines may be seen. Pain may be elicited through lateral compression of the plantar lesion but may also be painful on ambulation with direct pressure. If it involves the nail unit, the nail may become dystrophic from the pressure and presence of the lesion.

There are several treatments of verrucae; however, none of them is specific to HPV. They include use of keratolytic agents (salicylic acid), cryotherapy (liquid nitrogen), laser (pulsed dye and CO_2), bleomycin, candida antigen, and many home and folk remedies.

FUNGAL INFECTIONS

Superficial fungal infections, commonly known as ringworm, are mainly caused by dermatophytes that have been transmitted from human to human contact or by animal to human contact.[22] The most common dermatophytes seen are trichophyton, epidermophyton, and microsporum. Of these, *Trichophyton rubrum* is the most common pathogen. In addition to the dermatophytes, *Candida albicans* and nondermatophyte molds may play a role in these skin conditions. Diagnostic tests to determine a presence of a dermatophyte are a KOH test, periodic acid–Schiff stain, and fungal culture. If a pustule or more unusual presentation of these infections is present, a biopsy may be warranted.

Tinea Capitis

In children, a flaky and dry scalp should be considered tinea capitis until proved otherwise. Areas of staphylococcus superinfection around hair follicles are termed *kerion*. Oral griseofulvin remains a standard treatment in tinea capitis.

Tinea Pedis

The most common dermatophyte infection occurs on the feet in 1 of 3 formations: moccasin type, interdigital type, and vesicular type. The interdigital type is thought to be caused by the combination of excessive moisture breaking down the skin barrier, which allows the dermatophyte colonizing fomites (such as in shoes, showers, and carpets) to invade. This scaly rash typically presents in the fourth interdigital interspace as a scale with slight maceration. Patients may or may not have pruritus, erythema, or burning associated with the skin involvement.

The moccasin type presents as serpiginous scale that extends from the plantar aspect of the foot to the junction of the dorsal and plantar skin. Erythrema and pruritus may or may not be present. The vesicular type is an eczematous or inflammatory reaction pattern of the presence of the dermatophyte on the skin, which presents as small vesicles or pustules on the plantar aspect of the foot or on the dorsal aspect of the skin near the site of interdigital tinea. Pustular psoriasis, allergic contact dermatitis (ACD), and dyshidrotic eczema should be ruled out.

Topical antifungal medications are the first line of treatment along with education of proper personal hygiene (drying well in-between toes after bathing and wearing moisture-wicking socks); however, a mild lactic acid moisturizer may be added to help descale any dry areas. In addition, silver-treated fabric socks act that as an antimicrobial and 5-fingered socks to separate digits and keep topical medications in place may be considered.[23]

Tinea Incognito

Tinea incognito may occur after inappropriately placing an extremely potent topical corticosteroid on a fungal infection. At first, the topical steroid masks the fungal infection as inflammation and other symptoms decrease. Once the topical steroid is withdrawn, the quiescent fungal infection flares and flourishes. At this point, the appropriate topical antifungal should be applied and the topical steroid discontinued.

Onychomycosis

Tinea unguium, or onychomycosis, is dermatophyte infection of the nail unit. Clinically, it may be difficult to distinguish onychomycosis from the other existing nail pathologies. KOH preparation, periodic acid–Schiff staining, and fungal culture aid in determining the presence of a dermatophyte-caused infection. There are several types recognized by their initial site of involvement and pathophysiology. The classification of onychomycosis is as follows.[24]

Distal (or distal lateral) subungual
Distal (or distal lateral) subungual onychomycosis is the most common type in children and presents as onycholysis, discoloration, subungual debris, and hyperkeratosis. Concurrent tinea pedis is often seen interdigitally or plantarly on the foot. *Trichophyton rubrum* is the most common pathogen.[24]

Proximal subungual
The proximal subungual onychomycosis variety is not common but can occur in children. It is commonly seen in immunocompromised patients as a leukonychia, or white discoloration of the proximal nail plate. Distal subungual debris is generally not seen in this manifestation. *Trichophyton rubrum* and nondermatophyte molds are the common pathogens in this nail disease.

Candidal
Onychomycosis caused by candida is most often observed in patients who have chronic mucocutaneous candidiasis. The nail presents with onycholysis and paronychia. Total dystrophic onychomycosis, where the entire nail unit is infected and is caused by candida, is not often seen in the pediatric population.

Superficial white
The white powdery material seen in the superficial white type of onychomycosis is present on the dorsal aspect of the nail plate and could be scraped off with a scalpel blade. It is seen in tropical climates and is typically caused by *Trichophyton mentagrophytes* or nondermatophyte molds. Proximal subungual onychomycosis may be mistakenly identified as superficial white in very young children due to their thin nail plates.[24]

Management of onychomycosis includes débridement, topical ciclopirox, oral griseofulvin, and oral terbinafine in a weight-based dosage. Topical urea preparations of varying strengths may also be used to decrease the thickness of the nail plate.

Candidiasis

Candida albicans itself is a natural part of the skin flora. Conditions, such as antibiotic use, diabetes, obesity, immunosuppresion, and systemic steroid use, can cause candida to become more than just a natural skin colonizer. Candida infections usually occur in moist, intertriginous areas, such as the interdigital web spaces. Nail folds may also be affected, which causes a lifting of the eponychium and edema of the surrounding periungual tissue. If candidiasis occurs in these conditions, treatment of the malady helps, but often a topical steroid or topical antifungal belonging to the imidazole class provides relief.

ECZEMA/DERMATITIS
Overview

The terms, *eczema* and *dermatitis*, are interchangeable terms that refer to an inflammatory condition of the skin. Common skin signs of inflammation are calor (heat), rubor (redness), tumor (swelling), and pruritus (itching), which ultimately point to skin barrier dysfunction. The skin barrier, which is stratum corneum with the lipid-enriched extracellular matrix surrounding the corneocytes, is the body's protective wall and regulates homeostasis and transepidermal water loss (TEWL) and prevents entry of foreign particles and pathogens into the body. In general, eczema is characterized as having acute, subacute, and chronic phases, which are caused by either exogenous or endogenous conditions. During the acute phase, patients experience intense pruritus with an erythematous scaling and oozing skin rash with or without vesicles. Histologically, this is seen as epidermal intercellular edema or spongiosis as well as perivascular infiltrate of lymphocytes, macrophages, and eosinophils in the dermis. Clinically, this can also appear as dry skin eczema, contact dermatitis, stasis dermatitis, or even a dermatophyte infection. Subacute forms of atopic dermatitis present as a less intense pruritic, erythematous, scaling, and fissured skin rash. Chronic eczema presents with pruritus, hyperpigmented and hypopigmented well-defined plaques of previous inflamed skin, scales, and lichenification; this represents a hypertrophied epidermis.

Endogenous Eczema

Atopic dermatitis
The most common eczematous reaction seen is atopic dermatitis (AD), which affects up to 15% to 30% of children.[25] This chronic, relapsing disease is usually inherited, because patients present with a personal or family history of asthma, allergic rhinitis, eosinophilic esophagitis, or skin rash appropriate for their age. It is often described as an "itch that gets a rash," which is intensely pruritic, and cannot be described as having a primary lesion, as is the case with psoriasis and lichen planus. Although the cause is unknown, development of AD is a complex relationship of genetics, environment, and immune factors, which can lead to a negative quality of life and economically burden a pediatric patient's family. Patients with atopic eczema present with total immunoglobulin E elevation and sensitivity to environmental allergens, but the advent of identifying mutations in the stratum corneum protein filaggrin has shifted the focus to maintaining the skin barrier as a means of managing the disease.[25] It has been shown that these specific filaggrin mutations increase a greater risk of developing severe eczema in children as well as the development of airway disease in those same affected patients.[26]

Atopic eczema can present as 3 stages: infants (below the age of 2) tend to develop the lesions on the face and scalp with crusted, impetiginized lesions secondarily occurring while sparing the diaper area; children develop lesions on the flexural surfaces, dorsum of the limbs, and the nape of the neck; adolescents and adults present with lichenified lesions on the face, neck, and flexural surfaces[25]; 60% of the cases clear by adolescence; however, some go onto adulthood with a chronic, relapsing skin condition.[27]

Juvenile plantar dermatosis (sweaty sock dermatitis)
Exclusively seen in children and adolescents, juvenile plantar dermatosis (sweaty sock dermatitis), a dry, pink, and shiny skin condition, occurs bilaterally on the weight-bearing surface of the forefoot while sparing the interdigital areas.[28] Over time, fissuring may occur, making ambulation painful and difficult. It is thought to occur

more frequently in the winter, but a child playing and sweating in socks and shoes all day, removing them at night to dry, and continuing that wet-and dry-cycle daily contributes to this condition. It is frequently misdiagnosed as tinea pedis and atopic dermatitis and is recalcitrant to therapies associated with those conditions. Erythema and pruritus are rarely present and a new routine of foot hygiene must be implemented, including frequent changing of socks and shoes, wearing open-toed shoes, cleansing of the feet once shoes have been removed, and application of a barrier-restoring moisturizer if needed. Overall, this condition usually spontaneously resolves by age 14.

Pompholyx (dyshidrotic eczema)

Pompholyx is a chronic, relapsing eczematous reaction that is characterized by spongiosis and edema of the epidermis of both the palms and/or the soles. It is not solely due to excessive sweating as its name implies but can be aggravated by hyperhidrosis, emotional stress, occlusion, tinea pedis, and nickel. In children, it might be seen in addition to AD whereas in adults it might be seen with occupational hand dermatitis.[29] It can be pruritic and difficult to distinguish from other dermatoses but has been classically described as multiple tiny vesicles that are deep seated around the digits and may coalesce to form larger bullae. Pruritus may or may not be involved and, in general, is difficult to treat. Classic treatment options have included a combination of topical and systemic therapies depending on the severity: topical and systemic steroids, potassium permanganate soaks to prevent secondary staphylococcus infection, and aluminum acetate soaks to desiccate. Newer agents used to treat this condition include topical calcineurin inhibitors to decrease inflammation, botulinum toxin type A injections to decrease hyperhidrosis, topical retinoids, and phototherapy (psoralen–UV-A irradiation).

Exogenous Eczema/Dermatitis

Allergic contact dermatitis

ACD is an eczematous skin reaction that occurs after 1 or more exposures to a potential allergen. The reaction may take anywhere from 14 to 21 days to manifest and is termed *cell-mediated delayed hypersensitivity reaction*. Skin manifestation of ACD is as described previously, with acute, subacute, and chronic stages at the initial point of contact or may wander with further skin on skin contact. Its documentation in the pediatric population has increased due to diagnosis of AD and patch testing more frequently. During the pediatric patient initial visit, a detailed environmental history should include personal products used (shampoo, soap, diaper balms and wipes, and lotions); any medications used currently and previously; and parental/home products, such as detergent, cleansers, toys, play mats, and pets. In patients with atopic dermatitis that is chronic, severe, and not responding to the typical therapeutic agents, a diagnosis of ACD should be entertained. Children with new-onset dermatitis or those whose skin condition is spreading to other body sites and also do not have a personal or family history of atopy (asthma, allergic rhinitis, or skin disease) should also be patch tested.[30] Although some practitioners are concerned that patch testing may precipitate ACD, patch testing in the pediatric population should include the most common allergens seen: nickel, cobalt, neomycin/antibiotics, fragrance, and rubber.[30] Once the allergen has been identified, an avoidance regimen of the aggravator should be instituted.

Irritant contact dermatitis

Unlike ACD, irritant contact dermatitis (ICD) usually occurs in all cases where the chemical is exposed to the skin. An irritant, such as a caustic acid or alkali, provides instant damage to the epithelial cells and does not require prior sensitization. Examples of common irritants are soaps, detergents, and chlorine in swimming pools. In infants, it is common to see ICD in the diaper area due to exposure of stool and urine and to maceration and friction from the diaper itself.[31] Skin reaction is generally limited to the point of contact and is more severe with longer exposure of the irritant. As with ACD, once the aggravator has been identified, avoidance needs to be maintained by the patient.

Focus on Eczema/Dermatitis of the Lower Extremity

A blistering, erythematous inflamed skin rash presenting on the lower extremity in pediatric patients generally is seen on the dorsum of the foot and anterior aspect of the legs that may or may not be symmetric. If there is a blistering dermatitis of the plantar aspect of the feet, vesicular tinea pedis, pustular psoriasis, pompholyx, AD, and ACD must be considered. If a patient is experiencing the chronic stage of eczema, fissures and dry skin may be present at the dorsoplantar junction of the heel and peridigital area.

General Management of Eczema

With the advent of focusing on the epidermal barrier as problematic in eczematous skin, a paradigm shift has occurred. The first focus should be on improving the skin barrier with moisturizers, emollients, and ceramide-based creams. These creams decrease TEWL, which enhances the function of the epidermal skin barrier. The second is decreasing inflammation and itching with the gold standard as topical corticosteroids but now also includes topical calcineurin inhibitors for the steroid-phobic, weak responders to topical corticosteroids and facial use. Third, preventing infection in these patients is paramount because *Staphylococcus aureus* colonization and possible pathogenic involvement in atopic dermatitis patients has been documented.[32] *Staphylococcus aureus* can be isolated from 90% of skin lesions in atopic dermatitis[33] when it is rarely found on healthy skin. Oral antibiotics, topical antibiotics, antibacterial soaps, and bath additives and dressings have all been used with varying success. For example, the use of dilute bleach baths (concentration of 0.005%) with periodic intranasal application of mupirocin ointment was found to decrease the disease severity in those who frequently develop staphylococcus superinfections.[23] Avoiding triggers in these patients involves identifying food allergies, airborne allergies (pet dander and dust), and, in cases of ACD, the offending allergens. Also, changing body and laundry soap to mild fragrance-free preparations without the addition of bleach or fabric softeners can be useful. Cotton clothing should be worn with the avoidance of wool or rough fabrics. If cotton fabric is still too rough for a child, a randomized controlled study consisting of patients wearing silk fabric (DermaSilk) coated with an antimicrobial substance (AEM 5572/5) improved the symptoms of AD versus wearing cotton, and another study showed the silk-treated fabric was comparable to treatment with a topical steroid.[34] Finally, if external environment is a trigger for a patient, severe heat and low humidity should be avoided.

PSORIASIS
Plaque Psoriasis

In general, psoriasis is a T-cell–mediated inflammatory skin condition. Approximately 70% of children develop plaque psoriasis, which presents as an erythematous plaque with a silvery scale.[35] These lesions are geographic, bilateral, and symmetric, typically occurring on the extensor surfaces and scalp. The plaques can also be pruritic and affect joints as well as the nails during the progression of the disease. The diaper area can be involved in infancy and regress there as the child develops. ICD, ACD, and candidiasis must be ruled out in the diaper area. If psoriasis develops during childhood, there is a genetic link, with HLA-Cw6 the susceptible gene. Other characteristics associated with plaque psoriasis are the Koebner phenomenon, which is presence of the plaque in areas of trauma; the Auspitz sign, which is bleeding on scratching of the lesion; and pitting of the nail plate.

Pustular Psoriasis

Besides plaque psoriasis, pustular psoriasis can appear as sterile pustules on the plantar foot and palm of the hand. The pustules are visible forms of the Munro microabscesses, and varying stages of the lesion are generally seen on the same skin surface. After the pustules form, they evolve into a golden amber color and then desquamate. Vesicular tinea pedis and pompholyx must be ruled out.

Guttate Psoriasis

Most commonly after a streptococcus throat infection, guttate psoriasis appears as small salmon-colored plaques on the trunk, abdomen, and back. It is seen more in the pediatric population than adults. The group A β-hemolytic streptococcus does not cause the psoriasis; instead, the body's own inflammatory response is thought the causative factor.

Focus on Psoriasis of the Lower Extremity

Plantar plaque and pustular psoriasis are frequently misdiagnosed as either vesicular or moccasin tinea pedis. Due to the fissuring that often accompanies psoriatic plaques, they also are misdiagnosed as xerosis. If a patient's current treatment consists of either an oral or topical antifungal and is not improving the skin condition within the appropriate time frame, a biopsy of the skin to determine if a topical steroid should be used is warranted. On examination of the lower extremity, the hands should also be examined for involvement to diagnose palmoplantar psoriasis. Also, if a patient only presents with an onychomycosis-like nail involvement and has failed oral antifungals, a diagnosis of psoriatic nail disease should be considered. Another clue to aid in the diagnosis of psoriatic nails includes examining for the presence of erythema periungually, onycholysis, and pitting. Patients may also present with the arthritic component of psoriasis, which may manifest in dactylitis of the digits (sausage toes), enthesitis of the Achilles tendon, and distal interphalangeal joint involvement.

General Management of Psoriasis

Psoriasis not only is a disease of the skin, nails, and joints but also affects patients psychosocially. In addition, recent reports in adults have linked it to the metabolic syndrome, where sufferers of the disease are more likely to develop a cardiac event.[36] Even with all these comorbidities, a single treatment to resolve the disease has not been elucidated. As discussed previously, it is a chronic, relapsing disease that flares not only in times of stress and illness but also idiopathically. Older topical therapies like tar, anthralin, and salicylic acid are still used, but the gold standard is topical corticosteroids. Low potencies of topical corticosteroids are used for the face and interdigital areas, whereas midpotency formulations are used for the body and extremities. Injecting triamcinolone into the nail matrix is one way of treating psoriatic toenail disease. Concern for the side effects of the topical steroids has warranted the use of topical calcipotriene and calcitriol and topical calcineurin inhibitors. As with patients with AD, physicians should encourage use of the skin barrier moisturizers and repair creams to decrease TEWL. Phototherapy can also be considered in pediatric patients, namely, narrowband UV-B and psoralen–UV-A. Systemic therapies have included oral antibiotics, oral methotrexate, and oral cyclosporine and oral retinoids in more recalcitrant cases. The advent of injectable and intravenous biologic therapies that are tumor necrosis factor α inhibitors, such as etanercept and infliximab, have offered new ways of targeting the inflammatory cascade.

NEVI

Congenital melanocytic nevi (CMN) are classified as lesions that present at birth to 1 year of age. These lesions extend deep into the dermis and enlarge along with a child's growth. They are classified as small (most common at <1.5 cm), medium (1.5–20 cm), and giant (>20 cm). These nevi may have an irregular border and have hair growing through them. The giant CMN have a lifetime chance of 5% to 10% of developing melanoma, especially in the first 5 years of life.[37] It is currently recommended to completely excise (after staged procedures) a giant CMN as early as possible to decrease the risk of melanoma. If excision is not possible, careful observation is warranted and application of other modalities, such as ablative laser or curettage of the lesion, may be used. The small and medium-sized lesions have a smaller risk of developing melanoma but may also be managed in a similar way—elective excision and cosmetic reduction via laser.

Acquired melanocytic nevi begin to appear after the first 6 months of life and may be classified as junctional, compound, or intradermal. The nests of melanocytes may rest at the dermoepidermal junction as in junctional nevi or may migrate deeper to the dermis as in intradermal nevi. As the melanocytes migrate, the nevi appear elevated and less pigmented clinically. Junctional nevi are macular in appearance; compound nevi are slightly elevated because they are a combination of the junctional and intradermal types; and intradermal nevi are elevated and often flesh colored. Overall, these acquired lesions appear symmetric, evenly pigmented from a deep brown to tan color, and well defined.[37] Acquired melanocytic nevi arise from a combination of environment (sun exposure) and genetics.

Acral nevi present on the plantar aspect of the feet and may have pigmented streaks in them when viewed clinically or with a dermatoscope. This pattern reflects the dermatoglyphics of the plantar skin. Mostly macular, these lesions may also have a slightly raised appearance.

Atypical nevi are benign melanocytic lesions that clinically may overlap with the signs of melanoma (asymmetric, border notching, color variegation, and larger than 6 mm) but are different histologically from melanoma.[37] Because these lesions begin to appear in these children during puberty, it is imperative patients have periodic total body skin examinations that include a clinical examination, digital photography, and dermoscopy to determine which, if any, lesions require a skin biopsy.

Blue nevi are benign proliferations of active melanocytes that present as a blue to black papule on the dorsum of the hands and feet. These benign, solitary lesions may be confused with nodular melanoma and should be biopsied if there is a sudden change in appearance.

Commonly arising on the lower extremity and face during childhood, Spitz nevi are benign lesions that may have several characteristics that overlap histopathologically with melanoma. These symmetric, well-defined lesions can have a rapid growth phase and may appear as pink to red-brown papules and nodules. If there is any atypia clinically, these lesions should be excised completely during the initial biopsy.

Pediatric melanoma is rare and not easily defined with the adult ABCDs (A, asymmetry; B, border and bleeding; C, color; D, diameter; E, evolution) of melanoma guidelines. In a child who has multiple atypical nevi and is at greater risk of developing melanoma, the "ugly duckling" guide of observing a lesion that is not similar to the surrounding lesions may be useful when deciding whether to biopsy. In these children, it is helpful to determine personal and family history as well as observe risk factors (fair skin, freckles, and multiple sunburns) and recommend protective clothing and sunscreen. Childhood melanomas often are amelanotic and of the aggressive nodular type. They may mimic verrucae, scars, or vascular tumors. Once melanoma is diagnosed, sentinel lymph node biopsies and complete lymph node dissection can be explored, but the prognosis of these procedures has yet to be determined.[38]

NAILS

When considering nail disorders, practitioners should not be limited to disease caused by a dermatophyte. Practitioners should consider in the pediatric population nail changes caused by trauma, inflammation, infection, metabolic disorders, pigmentary disorders, and tumors. The most common issue seen in podopediatrics is paronychia of the great toenail, or inflammation of the lateral and proximal nail folds, usually accompanying an incurvated and ingrown, or onychocryptotic, nail plate. Purulence due to a *Staphylococcus aureus* infection is generally seen in this condition on the feet whereas candida infection is seen more in chronic thumbsuckers. Ingrown toenails with accompanying granulation tissue at the lateral nail fold are generally painful and can be malodorous. Treatment includes topical antibiotic and anti-inflammatory medications, oral antibiotic therapy, taping of the offending nail border to pull the inflamed skin away from the nail, education on proper nail trimming, incision and drainage of the abscess, and surgical removal of the onychocryptotic nail plate.

Onychomycosis, or tinea unguium, is caused by invasion of the nail unit by dermatophytes, nondermatophyte molds, and/or *Candida albicans*. Onychomycosis is seen in increasing amounts in the pediatric population, which is linked to juvenile diabetes and obesity.[39] Tinea pedis or tinea cruris on the child or parent may be concomitantly found. The most common form seen is distal lateral subungual caused by *Trichophyton rubrum*. Treatment includes oral griseofulvin, terbinafine (dosed for weight), and topical ciclopirox.

Trachyonychia is also referred to as 20-nail dystrophy, or rough nails.[40] It can be seen in association with lichen planus, psoriasis, alopecia areata, and AD. It may be misdiagnosed as onychomycosis if the underlying inflammatory condition causing trachyonychia is not elucidated. Treatment includes filing or buffing of the nails, oral biotin supplements, urea nail preparations, and triamcinolone injections into the nail matrix. It may also spontaneously resolve with time.

Longitudinal melanonychia, or a longitudinal darkly pigmented band, can be seen on the nail plate. Its causes include trauma, melanocytic nevus, lentigo, fungal infection, metabolic disorders, and melanoma (rarely in children).

REFERENCES

1. McGrath JA, Eady RAJ, Pope FM. Anatomy and organization of human skin. Chapter 3. In: Burns T, Breathnach S, Cox N, et al, editors. Rook's textbook of dermatology, vol. 1. 7th edition. Oxford (United Kingdom): Wiley-Blackwell; 2004. p. 1–84.
2. Rothman KF. Minimizing the pain of office procedures in children. Curr Opin Pediatr 1995;7:415–22.

3. Uman LS, Chambers CT, McGrath PJ, et al. Psychological interventions for needle-based procedural pain and distress in children and adolescents. Cochrane Database Syst Rev 2006;(4):CD005179.
4. Duarte AM. Environmental skin injuries in children. Curr Opin Pediatr 1995;7: 423–30.
5. Almahameed A, Pinto DS. Pernio (chilblains). Curr Treat Options Cardiovasc Med 2008;10(2):128–35.
6. Golant A, Nord RM, Paksima N, et al. Cold exposure injuries to the extremities. J Am Acad Orthop Surg 2008;16:704–15.
7. Heggers JP, Robson MC, Manavalen K, et al. Experimental and clinical observations on frostbite. Ann Emerg Med 1987;16(9):1056–62.
8. Schexnayder SM, Schexnayder RE. Bites, stings, and other painful things. Pediatr Ann 2000;29(6):354–8.
9. Karthikeyan K. Treatment of scabies: newer perspectives. Postgrad Med J 2005; 81(951):7–11.
10. Paller AS. Scabies in infants and small children. Semin Dermatol 1993;12(1):3–8.
11. Leung AK, Robson WL. Human bites in children. Pediatr Emerg Care 1992;8: 255–7.
12. Mailler-Savage EA, Adams BB. Skin manifestations of running. J Am Acad Dermatol 2006;55(2):290–301.
13. Lambert WF. Skin signs of child abuse. Available at: http://www.medscape.org/viewarticle/432571_3. Accessed March 22, 2016.
14. Braun-Falco M. Hereditary palmoplantar keratodermas. J Dtsch Dermatol Ges 2009;7:971–84.
15. Rapprich S, Hagedorn M. Surgical treatment of severe palmoplantar keratoderma. J Dtsch Dermatol Ges 2011;9(3):252–5.
16. Vayalumkal JV, Jadavji T. Children hospitalized with skin and soft tissue infections: a guide to antibacterial selection and treatment. Paediatr Drugs 2006;8: 99–111.
17. Palit A, Inamadar AC. Current concepts in the management of bacterial skin infections in children. Indian J Dermatol Venereol Leprol 2010;76(5):476–88.
18. Fiorillo L, Zucker M, Sawyer D, et al. The pseudomonas Hot-foot syndrome. N Engl J Med 2001;345:335–8.
19. Folster-Holst R, Kreth HW. Viral Exanthems in childhood—infectious (direct) exanthems. Part 1: classic exanthems. J Dtsch Dermatol Ges 2009;7(4):309–16.
20. Folster-Holst R, Kreth HW. Viral Exanthems in childhood—infectious (direct) exanthems. Part 2: other viral exanthems. J Dtsch Dermatol Ges 2009;7(5):414–9.
21. Mathes EF, Frieden IJ. Treatment of molluscum contagiosum with cantharidin: a practical approach. Pediatr Ann 2010;39(3):124–31.
22. Andrews RM, McCarthy J, Carapetis JR, et al. Skin disorders including pyoderma, scabies, and tinea infections. Pediatr Clin North Am 2009;56:1421–40.
23. Gelmetti C, Frasin A, Restano L. Innovative therapeutics in pediatric dermatology. Dermatol Clin 2010;28:619–29.
24. Gupta AK, Skinner AR, Baran R. Onychomycosis in children: an overview. J Drugs Dermatol 2003;2:31–4.
25. Beiber T. Atopic dermatitis. N Engl J Med 2008;358:1483–94.
26. Rodriguez E, Baurecht H, Herberich E, et al. Meta-analysis of filaggrin polymorphisms in eczema and asthma: robust risk factors in atopic disease. J Allergy Clin Immunol 2009;123(6):1361–70.
27. Williams HC. Atopic dermatitis: new information from epidemiological studies. Br J Hosp Med 1994;52(8):409–12.

28. Jones SK, English JS, Forsyth A, et al. Juvenile plantar dermatosis – an 8-year follow-up of 102 patients. Clin Exp Dermatol 1987;12:5–7.
29. Wollina W. Pompholyx: what's new? Expert Opin Investig Drugs 2008;17(6): 897–904.
30. Jacob SE, Burk CJ, Connelly EA. Patch Testing: another steroid-sparing agent to consider in children. Pediatr Dermatol 2008;25(1):81–7.
31. Alberta L, Sweeney SM, Wiss K. Diaper dye dermatitis. Pediatrics 2005;116: e450–2.
32. Birnie AJ, Bath-Hextall FJ, Ravenscroft JC, et al. Interventions to reduce Staphylococcus aureus in the management of atopic eczema: an updated Cochrane review. Br J Dermatol 2011;154(1):228.
33. Leyden JJ, Marples RR, Kligman AM. Staphylococcus aureus in the lesions of atopic dermatitis. Br J Dermatol 1974;90(5):525–30.
34. Senti G, Steinmann LS, Fischer B, et al. Antimicrobial silk clothing in the treatment of atopic dermatitis proves comparable to topical corticosteroid treatment. Dermatology 2006;213:228–33.
35. Silverberg NB. Pediatric psoriasis: an update. Ther Clin Risk Manag 2009;5: 849–56.
36. Gisondi P, Ferrazzi A, Girolomoni G. Metabolic comorbidities and psoriasis. Acta Dermatovenerol Croat 2010;18(4):297–304.
37. Schaffer JV. Pigmented lesions in children: when to worry. Curr Opin Pediatr 2007;19:430–40.
38. Kirkwood JM, Jukic D, Averbook BJ, et al. Melanoma in pediatric, adolescent, and young adult patients. Semin Oncol 2009;36(5):419–31.
39. Kwong PC. Dermatological issues in a child with diabetes mellitus. In: Menon RK, Sperling MA, editors. Pediatric diabetes. Norwell, MA: Kluwer Academic Publishers; 2003. p. 433.
40. Tosti A, Piraccini BM, Iorizzo M. Trachyonychia and related disorders: evaluation and treatment plans. Dermatol Ther 2002;15(2):121–5.

Importance of Vehicles in Topical Treatment of Fungal Infections

Leon H. Kircik, MD[a,b,c,]*

KEYWORDS

- Vehicle • Topical • Antifungal • Adherence

KEY POINTS

- Compared with systemic treatment, topical drug delivery provides 2 notable benefits in the management of skin diseases. First, medication can be efficiently deposited directly to the site of disease activity, potentially optimizing therapeutic response. Second, topical drug application generally results in little to no plasma concentration of the active drugs.
- The issue of secondary formulations may have therapeutic implications. Chemical and physical changes occur from the moment a formulation is applied to skin. For example, if a water-insoluble active molecule is formulated into an aqueous vehicle, as the water evaporates on application, the active molecule and its solvent are left on the skin, providing a higher effective concentration of active.
- Certain dosage forms may be better suited for use at certain anatomic sites. For example, an ointment is not ideal for application to the hairy scalp. Another consideration is the spreadability of a formulation.
- Of particular relevance to podiatric medicine, the emergence of topical treatments for toenail onychomycosis represents an especially interesting development in new vehicle formulation.
- A combination of 3 primary considerations may influence the selection of a particular topical formulation in the clinical setting: (1) anticipated efficacy; (2) supportive effects of the vehicle formulation; and (3) practical, patient-based considerations.

Topical drug therapies are commonly used to manage dermatologic diseases and their manifestations in the skin, hair, nails, and mucous membranes. Compared with systemic treatment, topical drug delivery provides 2 notable benefits in the management of skin diseases. First, medication can be efficiently deposited directly to the site of disease activity, potentially optimizing therapeutic response. Second, topical drug

Disclosure: Dr L.H. Kircik has received funding as an investigator, consultant, or advisory board member from Valeant, Merz, Pharmaderm, and Exeltis.

[a] Indiana University School of Medicine, Indianapolis, IN, USA; [b] Mount Sinai Medical Center, New York, NY, USA; [c] Physicians Skin Care, PLLC, 1169 Eastern Parkway, Suite 2310, Louisville, KY 40202, USA
* Physicians Skin Care, PLLC, 1169 Eastern Parkway, Suite 2310, Louisville, KY 40217.
E-mail address: wedoderm@yahoo.com

application generally results in little to no plasma concentration of the active drug, hence it is associated with low risk for systemic exposure and associated potential systemic side effects.

The modern pharmacologic landscape offers several topical dosage forms and many formulation bases, each with its own potential benefits. In many cases, the same active drug is available in several different dosage forms (**Box 1**), offering pre-scribers the ability to tailor treatment to the patient's unique presentation and needs. In the clinical setting, prescribers must identify the topical drug formulation that is best suited to the presentation of the disease and most likely to encourage therapeutic adherence. This process is best done with an understanding of topical drug delivery, vehicle formulation, and patient behaviors.

TOPICAL DRUG DELIVERY BASICS

Most topically applied drugs are metabolized in the epidermis. The enzyme-rich skin is the largest drug metabolizing organ. Biotransformation of compounds often occurs in the epidermis, presenting both challenges and opportunities to formulators. Epidermal biotransformation could render a drug ineffective before it reaches its target or, in the case of some prodrugs, synthesize a biologically inactive molecule to an active form.[1]

Although topical drug application seems intuitive in the management of dermato-logic diseases, topical drug delivery is no easy task. The epidermal barrier serves an important function: it prevents entry of chemicals, allergens, and other toxic elements into the body because these are all perceived as foreign bodies, including drugs.[2] Because of the action of the epidermal barrier and its general efficiency, the amount of topical drug that bypasses the epidermal barrier and is absorbed by the skin is typically minimal. This barrier function remains the case, even though impair-ment of epidermal barrier function is a characteristic of many common dermatoses.[3] The barrier is frequently impaired enough to cause symptoms or allow entry of path-ogens, but not enough to facilitate drug delivery.

Faced with this reality, topical drug formulators must engineer delivery vehicles that either bypass or override the barrier. This engineering may be done in various ways, and the approach depends to large extent on the active agent to be delivered. Char-acteristics such as the size, charge, solubility, and lipophilic or hydrophilic nature of the molecule influence the development process, with the ultimate goal of developing

---

Box 1
Topical dosage forms

Eight topical dosage forms recognized by the US Food and Drug Administration (FDA)

Solution

Suspension

Lotion

Paste

Gel

Ointment

Cream

Other (includes foams, aerosols, powders, patches, and so forth)

a formulation that effectively deposits the active drug, delivers it to the site of metabolism, and allows the drug to remain at the site long enough to render an effect (**Fig. 1**).

A well-designed vehicle should deposit the drug on the skin with even distribution and deliver the drug into the skin. However, the role of the vehicle does not end with drug transport; the vehicle must separate itself from the drug, permitting the drug to work at its intended site. At this stage, the vehicle itself may also offer supportive effects on the skin, such as occlusion or moisturizing. Note that occlusion may affect the bioavailability of a drug. For example, occlusion has been shown to increase the bioavailability of topically applied corticosteroids.[4] Many dermatologists conceptualize the effects of occlusion as akin to increasing the potency class in the case of steroids. In order to bypass the epidermal barrier, many drugs are delivered through combinations of transcellular, intercellular, and follicular absorption.[5]

Penetration-enhancing agents are commonly used in topical drug formulations to interrupt the barrier and facilitate drug delivery through the epidermis. The skin irritant propylene glycol is a common ingredient in topical formulations and, at high concentrations, is known to promote desquamation,[6,7] thus widening the intercellular pathways through which topically applied drugs may pass. Of the many solubilizing agents used, propylene glycol is probably best known and is perhaps associated with misconceptions. At high levels, propylene glycol is highly irritating to the skin. Propylene glycol may cause adverse skin reactions even at 2% concentration in patients with dermatitis.[8] Nonetheless, propylene glycol is generally well tolerated at lower concentrations, is commonly used in many topical drug formulations, and is the main excipient in most generic formulations, especially of corticosteroids.

Because of negative associations with the use of penetration enhancers, vehicle formulators have sought novel alternatives to enhance drug absorption. However, use of penetration enhancers remains necessary and is common. Ideally, formulations use only low concentrations of enhancers in concert with other tactics to encourage drug absorption. However, some formulations rely on high concentrations of enhancers, which may be the case with many generic topical corticosteroid formulations, as discussed later.[2]

Hydration of the stratum corneum is an alternative mode for modifying drug delivery. As epidermal cells swell, the aqueous/lipid ratio within the skin are altered; those cells no longer resist mechanical sheering and stress forces and allow entry of foreign molecules.[9]

Considerations in Topical Drug Development

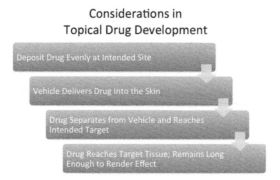

Deposit Drug Evenly at Intended Site

Vehicle Delivers Drug Into the Skin

Drug Separates from Vehicle and Reaches Intended Target

Drug Reaches Target Tissue; Remains Long Enough to Render Effect

Fig. 1. There are 4 primary considerations that drive vehicle formulation.

In addition to penetration enhancers, vehicle bases include other excipients, including possibly preservatives and skin conditioners, such as emollients, humectants, and occlusives. Recently, formulators have focused on strategies to counter the negative effects of penetration enhancers or drugs. Incorporating humectants like glycerin can enhance stratum corneum hydration. Emollients like dimethicone help improve the texture and feel of the skin and provide a temporary barrier to transepidermal water loss (TEWL).

Among excipients, fragrances or more likely masking agents may be added to formulations, either to provide a pleasant scent or to cover an unpleasant odor, thus allowing an unscented claim. The presence of fragrance may be clinically relevant, because fragrance contact allergy is highly prevalent in North America and Europe.[10] As such, prescribers should pay attention to the presence of fragrance or other potential allergens in a formulation.

The use of microspheres is an increasingly popular approach to minimize active drug-induced irritation. Slow release of active drugs through microspheres has been shown to reduce irritation and minimize the rate or percutaneous absorption.[11,12]

Secondary Formulations

The issue of secondary formulations is not frequently studied, although it may have therapeutic implications. Discussion of vehicle formulations almost always focuses on the primary formulation: what is contained within a tube, bottle, tub, or jar when it leaves the manufacturing line. However, chemical and physical changes occur from the moment a formulation is applied to the skin. For example, a water-insoluble active molecule may be formulated into a vehicle base with a high concentration of water. As the water evaporates on application, the active molecule and its solvent are left on the skin, providing a higher effective concentration of active than in the primary formulation. For example, an ethanolic foam formulation of clobetasol propionate was designed to form a supersaturated secondary formulation following application to the skin. As the alcohol component of the foam evaporates, the concentration of active drug in the residual formulation is effectively increased.

THE DOSAGE FORM

Ensuring chemical delivery of the active drug is crucial; however, the clinical efficacy of any treatment depends on its proper use. The dosage form may have a direct influence on therapeutic adherence and, therefore, on therapeutic outcomes.[13] However, adherence rates in developed countries may be as low as 50%.[14]

Many of the terms commonly used to describe specific vehicles derive from marketing departments and do not reflect officially recognized vehicle bases. The 8 topical dosage forms recognized by the US Food and Drug Administration (FDA) are:

- Solution
- Suspension
- Lotion
- Paste
- Gel
- Ointment
- Cream
- Other (includes foams, aerosols, powders, patches, and so forth)[15]

A recent study investigated patient preferences for topical formulations across numerous dermatologic diseases. Researchers found strong preference for formulations that were, "moisturizing, absorbs/disappears/dries quickly, available in various formulations, does not bleach or stain skin/hair/clothing, is not greasy or oily, is not sticky or tacky, is long lasting/long acting, is fragrance or odor free, is easy to apply/simple to use, and can use all the time."[14]

Certain dosage forms may be better suited for use at certain anatomic sites. For example, an ointment is not ideal for application to the hairy scalp. In contrast, a foam formulation may be especially suited for use on large body surfaces or on hair-bearing areas. Another consideration is the spreadability of a formulation. On painful, irritated skin, patients may prefer the ease of application of a foam or gel, compared with the manipulation needed to apply an ointment.

The first foam vehicles on the market contained ethanol, which has drying effects. Next-generation foams incorporate emollients. These emollients dissolve at body temperature, collapsing the foam. The emollients then lie on top of the skin providing hydration and a temporary barrier effect.[16]

First-generation alcohol-based gels are not widely used now because they were frequently drying and led to irritation. Instead, hydrogels have been developed that have a high water content but no acetone, alcohol, or significant levels of harsh solvents. In studies, the water-based hydrogel vehicle has been shown to improve skin hydration and not further impair epidermal barrier function (as indicated by TEWL).[17] Patient acceptance of this base is high. In one study, 100% of subjects said that they found a hydrogel formulation of topical corticosteroid to be easy to apply/use/spread, easy to use on hair-bearing skin, comfortable to use under makeup and/or cosmetics, suitable for use on multiple body areas, and stain free.[18]

Of particular relevance to podiatric medicine, the emergence of topical treatments for toenail onychomycosis represents an especially interesting development in new vehicle formulation. Ciclopirox first-generation toenail lacquer had been seen as a welcome, although less-effective, alternative to systemic treatments.[19] A newer topical formulation, efinaconazole topical solution, 10%, is an effective and well-tolerated treatment of onychomycosis. It has been shown that efinaconazole results in greater cumulative nail penetration compared with ciclopirox.[20] The penetration and associated efficacy have been attributed to the low surface tension of the formulation, which affords better penetration of efinaconazole through the nail plate, and also to the site of infection by spreading into the space between the nail and nail bed.[21] Another new topical solution for onychomycosis, tavaborole, also shows good penetration. It has been shown to penetrate through the nail and up to 4 layers of cosmetic nail polish.[22]

Despite growth in the adoption of next-generation or nontraditional topical vehicles with documented patient care and therapeutic benefits, their use in clinical practice remains low, especially outside of dermatology.[23]

Knowledge of dosage forms can be relevant to understanding the development of generic challengers of innovator formulations. To apply for marketing approval from the FDA, a generic formulation must challenge a specific existing product (active drug, concentration, and dosage form). Although the active ingredient and its concentration are the same, the vehicle excipients may differ significantly between an innovator and a generic and between different generics. These formulation differences could manifest clinically in:

- Differences in treatment-associated irritancy
- Allergenicity
- Possibly in potency and efficacy, as further discussed later (**Box 2**)

Box 2
Vehicle affects potency

Example: betamethasone dipropionate 0.05%

Class I
   Diprolene cream, 0.05%
   Diprolene ointment, 0.05%

Class II
   Diprolene cream AF, 0.05%
   Diprosone ointment 0.05%

Class III
   Diprosone cream 0.05%

Class V
   Diprosone lotion 0.05%

The same active corticosteroid molecule can have a different potency class, depending on features of the vehicle formulation. Among the potential potency-influencing effects of a vehicle are occlusion and enhanced absorption of drug through the stratum corneum.

The prescription should not be substituted for different dosage forms or vehicles than the one prescribed by the provider, although this practice seems to be widespread.

TREATMENT SELECTION

A combination of 3 primary considerations may influence the selection of a particular topical formulation in the clinical setting. These are anticipated:

1. Efficacy
2. Supportive effects of the vehicle formulation
3. Practical, patient-based considerations

Anticipated Efficacy

Published clinical trial results offer a reasonable indication of a formulation's efficacy. As is well established, the controls of a clinical trial do not exist in real-world use, and clinical outcomes may vary in actual use. Factors like patient age and sex, adherence, and baseline disease severity can all modulate efficacy. Nonetheless, clinical trial data offer a reasonable basis for conceptualizing a drug's potential benefits and safety.

As a practical matter, there is no true placebo in topical treatment studies. The vehicle formulation exerts effects on the skin. In many studies of modern formulations, subjects in the vehicle-only groups have had notable improvements in the signs and symptoms of psoriasis, dermatitis, and other skin diseases. These findings show the beneficial skin-supporting effects of a well-designed vehicle.

One of the reasons many prescribers prefer branded formulations to generics is that these innovator formulations may offer more reliable trial data and consistent clinical performance. Generic topical formulations rarely publish efficacy figures and are not required to conduct clinical efficacy trials. Instead, generic products must show bioequivalence to the reference listed drug or innovator through simple tests, such as vasoconstrictor assays. If the generic formulation shows bioequivalence, it is assumed to have safety and efficacy equivalent to that of the innovator. Generic drugs may be considered bioequivalent if they are within a range of the innovator.

For example, for topical corticosteroids the FDA requires that the 90% confidence interval for the ratio of the area under the effect curve (AUEC) caused by the test product and the AUEC caused by the reference product does not differ significantly, this is defined as 20%. As such, the generic's bioequivalence could be as low as 80% or as high as 125% of the innovator.

Another difference between branded and generic formulations is in formulation consistency. A branded drug formulation has the same composition from batch to batch over time. Generic manufacturers have more latitude in modifying their formulations, substituting excipients or modifying their concentrations, often in order to manage production costs. Further, should the pharmacy change distributors or the patient switch pharmacies, the patient may obtain a different generic formulation than was previously used. This possibility may introduce a level of variability into therapy that can be up to 45%.

Supportive Effects

It is now accepted that the vehicle base does more than deliver a drug. It can support skin healing by offering beneficial effects on the epidermis and the barrier. In contrast, a poorly designed vehicle can have detrimental effects on the skin. Epidermal barrier dysfunction is common to many dermatoses, including dermatophytoses.[24] Barrier dysfunction may contribute to symptoms like itching and dryness and promote skin breakdown. Excipients in the vehicle like alcohol can not only encourage barrier disruption but may also cause stinging and burning. In contrast, emollients, lipids, and humectants may support barrier repair and help improve symptoms. With this knowledge in mind, prescribers must consider the secondary effects not only of the drug but also of the formulation.

Consider a novel formulation of the broad-spectrum antifungal econazole nitrate foam 1% for once-daily use (Ecoza, Exeltis). Results of 2 vehicle-controlled trials of interdigital tinea pedis treated with econazole nitrate foam 1% show that 24.3% of econazole-treated patients achieved complete cure (negative KOH test, negative fungal culture, complete resolution of all signs and symptoms), compared with 3.6% for foam vehicle. Subjects applied econazole or vehicle once daily for 4 weeks and were assessed at 2 weeks after their last treatment (day 43). Treated patients had higher rates of mycologic cure (67.6% vs 16.9%) and effective treatment (48.6% vs 10.8%) versus foam vehicle. Econazole nitrate foam 1% was safe and well tolerated; its safety profile was comparable with that of the foam vehicle. No serious adverse events were reported for econazole nitrate foam 1%.[25]

Ecoza is formulated with a patented Proderm Technology that may help to enhance drug delivery through the skin. Proderm is an alcohol-free vehicle base that contains a mixture of water and lipids, according to the manufacturer. These lipids are intended to help restore epidermal moisture, thus treatment enhances epidermal barrier repair because of the unique characteristics of the foam vehicle.

Practical Considerations

For hair-bearing skin, a spray, foam, or gel may be easier to apply than other vehicle bases. Foams and gels may dry quickly on the skin, which may, for example, make them suitable for application on the foot before putting on socks or shoes. In contrast, creams or ointments may leave a greasy skin residue that is not well tolerated in socks or shoes.

Solutions for treatment of onychomycotic toenails may provide a patient-friendly and convenient alternative to oral agents. When the application site is difficult to reach, such as the toes or palms of an elderly patient, patients may find a topical spray beneficial.

Dosing frequency is also key to consider. Luliconazole cream 1% is the first topical azole antifungal agent approved to treat tinea cruris and tinea corporis with a 1-week, once-daily treatment regimen. It is indicated for the topical treatment of interdigital tinea pedis, tinea cruris, and tinea corporis caused by *Trichophyton rubrum* and *Epidermophyton floccosum* in patients 18 years of age and older.

In a phase II study of luliconazole for the treatment of interdigital tinea pedis, complete clearance was achieved in 26.8% and 45.7% of subjects in the 2-week and 4-week treatment groups at 2 weeks posttreatment, respectively.[26] The antifungal effect persisted several weeks posttreatment, resulting in increased rates of mycologic and clinical cure. Four weeks posttreatment complete clearance rates were 53.7% and 62.9% for the 2-week and 4-week treatment groups, respectively.

In a comparison of in vitro and in vivo antidermatophyte activities, luliconazole showed strong antifungal activity against *Trichophyton* spp; its minimum inhibitory concentration was 1 to 4 times lower than that of lanoconazole or terbinafine.[27] Seven-day topical therapy with a 0.5% solution of luliconazole was more effective than lanoconazole or terbinafine (0.5%). Only luliconazole achieved complete mycologic cure.

Also available, Naftin (naftifine HCl, Merz North America) gel 2% for the treatment of interdigital-type tinea pedis offers a once-daily application treatment regimen. In clinical studies, Naftin gel 2% showed continuous improvement in posttreatment efficacy rates for up to 4 weeks after the treatment regimen had ended.

The persistent effect of these newer topical antifungal formulations seems to be related to the ability of the vehicle to effectively deliver active drug into various layers of the stratum corneum, as shown in tape strip studies.[28,29] The highest mean levels of naftifine chloride were recovered from the stratum corneum 3 days after the last dose was applied; at day 43, the level remained several orders of magnitude higher than on day 1.[28] In guinea pig models, topically applied luliconazole cream achieved high concentrations in the stratum corneum by day 3 of application and remained at these levels through 14 days.[29]

By rapidly achieving a depot effect, these newer formulations allow a shorter overall treatment duration. Deep delivery of active drug into the stratum corneum targets dermatophytes at various levels of the stratum corneum, whereas formulations with more superficial delivery may target only a proportion of dermatophytes; unaffected dermatophytes can reemerge and create a recurrence of symptoms.

SUMMARY

- Topical drug delivery can be efficient and reduces systemic drug exposure.
- It should also be convenient to the patient, and the availability of different dosage forms allows providers to match treatment to each patient's unique presentation and therapeutic needs.
- In the current topical pharmacologic environment, the formulation itself plays an important role in treatment outcomes.
- A well-designed vehicle ensures drug delivery while also supporting epidermal barrier function.
- Prescribers should be aware of the vehicle options available when they prescribe and should also ensure that patients receive the exact formulation they prescribed, and not a substitution.

Sidebar: encouraging adherence

Research shows that patient preferences can significantly influence treatment adherence, satisfaction, and ultimate outcomes. As a general rule, patients seem to prefer topical vehicle bases that are moisturizing and absorb quickly, whereas they eschew formulations that are greasy or oily, sticky or tacky.[13] In some instances, the prescriber may have only 1 dosage form available. When there are options, take the time to ask the patient about preferences. Make no assumptions.

A spray, foam, or gel may be ideally suited for treatment of wet, macerated tinea pedis, but some patients may prefer a cream or ointment. The old adage, "If it's wet dry it; if it's dry wet it," has long been abandoned. The key is to apply an effective drug that the patient will use.

Sidebar: a closer look at wash-off therapies

Short-contact therapy is still not widely used, but the concept has been proved to be effective. Medicated shampoos and washes commonly deliver insoluble, particulate drugs, such as ketoconazole, that are deposited in the follicular ostium. Researchers found that leaving a ketoconazole shampoo in place for a 5-minute application produced no better improvement in dandruff than did immediate rinsing.[30] Ketoconazole shampoo has been shown to be effective for treatment of dandruff, seborrheic dermatitis, and tinea versicolor.[31,32]

REFERENCES

1. Kircik LH, Bikowski JB. Vehicles matter. Supplement to Practical Dermatology. 2010;7(3):1–16.

2. Proksch E, Brandner JM, Jensen JM. The skin: an indispensable barrier. Exp Dermatol 2008;17(12):1063–72.

3. Stalder JF, Tennstedt D, Deleuran M, et al. Fragility of epidermis and its consequence in dermatology. J Eur Acad Dermatol Venereol 2014; 28(Suppl 4):1–18.

4. Sommer A, Veraart J, Neumann M, et al. Evaluation of the vasoconstrictive effects of topical steroids by laser-Doppler-perfusion-imaging. Acta Derm Venereol 1998;78(1):15–8.

5. Chourasia R, Jain SK. Drug targeting through pilosebaceous route. Curr Drug Targets 2009;10(10):950–67.

6. Lanigan RS, Cosmetic Ingredient Review Expert Panel. Final report on the safety assessment of PPG-11 and PPG-15 stearyl ethers. Int J Toxicol 2001; 20(Suppl 4):53–9.

7. Lanigan RS, Cosmetic Ingredient Review Expert Panel. Amended final report on the safety assessment of PPG-40 butyl ether with an addendum to include PPG-2, -4, -5, -9, -12, -14, -15, -16, -17, -18, -20, -22, -24, -26, -30, -33, -52, and -53 butyl ethers. Int J Toxicol 2001;20(Suppl 4):39–52.

8. Loden M. Role of topical emollients and moisturizers in the treatment of dry skin barrier disorders. Am J Clin Dermatol 2003;4(11):771–88.

9. Pierard GE, Goffin V, Hermanns-Le T, et al. Corneocyte desquamation. Int J Mol Med 2000;6(2):217–21.

10. Cheng J, Zug KA. Fragrance allergic contact dermatitis. Dermatitis 2014;25(5): 232–45.

11. Embil K, Nacht S. The Microsponge Delivery System (MDS): a topical delivery system with reduced irritancy incorporating multiple triggering mechanisms for the release of actives. J Microencapsul 1996;13(5):575–88.

12. Jelvehgari M, Siahi-Shadbad MR, Azarmi S, et al. The microsponge delivery system of benzoyl peroxide: preparation, characterization and release studies. Int J Pharm 2006;308(1–2):124–32.

13. Eastman WJ, Malahias S, Delconte J, et al. Assessing attributes of topical vehicles for the treatment of acne, atopic dermatitis, and plaque psoriasis. Cutis 2014;94(1):46–53.

14. Sabaté E. Adherence to long-term therapies—evidence for action, WHO. 2003. Available at: http://apps.who.int/medicinedocs/pdf/s4883e/s4883e.pdf. Accessed January 16, 2014. WHO1–211.

15. Buhse L, Kolinski R, Westenberger B, et al. Topical drug classification. Int J Pharm 2005;295:101–12.

16. Tamarkin D, Friedman D, Shemer A. Emollient foam in topical drug delivery. Expert Opin Drug Deliv 2006;3(6):799–807.

17. Kircik LH. Transepidermal water loss (TEWL) and corneometry with hydrogel vehicle in the treatment of atopic dermatitis: a randomized, investigator-blind pilot study. J Drugs Dermatol 2012;11(2):180–4.

18. Trookman NS, Rizer RL, Ho ET, et al. The importance of vehicle properties to patients with atopic dermatitis. Cutis 2011;88(Suppl 1):13–7.

19. Shemer A, Nathansohn N, Trau H, et al. Ciclopirox nail lacquer for the treatment of onychomycosis: an open non-comparative study. J Dermatol 2010;37(2):137–9.

20. Sugiura K, Hosaka S, Arakawa Y, et al. Unique properties of efinaconazole 10% solution, a new topical treatment for onychomycosis. American Academy of Dermatology 71st Annual Meeting. Miami, FL, March 1–4, 2013.

21. Kircik LH. Enhancing transungual delivery and spreading of efinaconazole under the nail plate through a unique formulation approach. J Drugs Dermatol 2014; 13(12):1457–61.

22. Vlahovic T, Merchant T, Chanda S, et al. In vitro nail penetration of tavaborole topical solution, 5%, through nail polish on ex vivo human fingernails. J Drugs Dermatol 2015;14(7):675–8.

23. Huang KE, Davis SA, Cantrell J, et al. Increasing use of non-traditional vehicles for psoriasis and other inflammatory skin conditions. Dermatol Online J 2014; 20(9).

24. Lee WJ, Kim JY, Song CH, et al. Disruption of barrier function in dermatophytosis and pityriasis versicolor. J Dermatol 2011;38(11):1049–53.

25. Elewski BE, Vlahovic TC. Econazole nitrate foam 1% for the treatment of tinea pedis: results from two double-blind, vehicle-controlled, phase 3 clinical trials. J Drugs Dermatol 2014;13(7):803–8.

26. Jarratt M, Jones T, Kempers S, et al. Luliconazole for the treatment of interdigital tinea pedis: a double blind vehicle controlled study. Cutis 2013;91:203–10.

27. Scher RK, Nakamura N, Tavakkol A. Luliconazole: a review of a new antifungal agent for the topical treatment of onychomycosis. Mycoses 2014;57(7):389–93.

28. Plaum S, Verma A, Fleischer AB Jr, et al. Detection and relevance of naftifine hydrochloride in the stratum corneum up to four weeks following the last application of naftifine cream and gel, 2%. J Drugs Dermatol 2013;12(9):1004–8.

29. Koga H, Nanjoh Y, Inoue K, et al. In vitro activities of antifungal drugs against clinical isolates of *Trichophyton tonsurans*. Nihon Ishinkin Gakkai Zasshi 2006; 47(4):299–304 [in Japanese].

30. Piérard-Franchimont C, Uhoda E, Loussouarn G, et al. Effect of residence time on the efficacy of antidandruff shampoos. Int J Cosmet Sci 2003;25(6):267–71.
31. Ive FA. An overview of experience with ketoconazole shampoo. Br J Clin Pract 1991;45(4):279–84.
32. Lange DS, Richards HM, Guarnieri J, et al. Ketoconazole 2% shampoo in the treatment of tinea versicolor: a multicenter, randomized, double-blind, placebo-controlled trial. J Am Acad Dermatol 1998;39(6):944–50.

Adverse Drug Reactions of the Lower Extremities

 CrossMark

Chris G. Adigun, MD

KEYWORDS

- Drug • Pigmentation • Edema • Hand-foot-syndrome • Paronychia
- Onychomadesis • Nail

KEY POINTS

- Adverse drug reactions (ADRs) are a common dermatologic problem, and may involve any area of the skin, skin appendages, and mucosa.
- There are several ADRs that specifically affect the lower extremities.
- The nail apparatus is particularly vulnerable to toxicity from medications. Depending on the part of the nail apparatus affected, different clinical findings are observed.
- Although venous hypertension and subsequent pooling of interstitial fluid caused by venous valve incompetence is the most common cause of lower extremity edema, several medications can induce this condition, and should be considered in any patient with new-onset lower extremity edema.
- Chemotherapy agents cause several problems in the skin of the lower extremities and the nails. Recognizing and managing these ADRs is important because they can impede patients' ability to perform activities of daily living and to ambulate.

Adverse drug reactions (ADRs) are a common cause of dermatologic consultation, involving 2 to 3 per 100 medical inpatients in the United States. Female patients are 1.3 to 1.5 times more likely to develop ADRs, except in children less than 3 years of age, among whom boys are more often affected.[1] Certain drugs are more frequent causes, including aminopenicillins, trimethoprim-sulfamethoxazole, and nonsteroidal antiinflammatory drugs (NSAIDs).[2] ADRs can involve any area of the skin; the appendages, including hair and nails; as well as mucosa.

In addition, certain hypersensitivity syndromes to medications characteristically occur in conjunction with either active or latent infection with human herpes virus (HHV)–6, HHV-7, Epstein-Barr virus, cytomegalovirus, and human immunodeficiency virus. HLA type may also increase an individual's risk for ADRs to certain medications. T cells, specifically T-helper 1 (Th1) cells, are the primary inducers of ADRs. Systemic viral infections are thought to have already activated the T cells in the skin, theoretically lowering their threshold for drug binding and thereby increasing the risk of ADRs.[3]

Pinehurst Skin Surgery Center, 289 Olmsted Boulevard, Suite 5, Pinehurst, NC 28374, USA
E-mail address: chris.adigun@gmail.com

Clin Podiatr Med Surg 33 (2016) 397–408
http://dx.doi.org/10.1016/j.cpm.2016.02.007
0891-8422/16/$ – see front matter © 2016 Elsevier Inc. All rights reserved.

A skin appendage of the lower extremity that is particularly vulnerable to drug-induced changes is the nail apparatus. In general, nail abnormalities caused by medications can present with a wide range of clinical manifestations. These abnormalities tend to be dose related, and resolve with withdrawal of the offending agent. Many nail changes are asymptomatic and are more of a cosmetic nuisance, whereas others cause intense pain and impair activities of daily living and ambulation[4] (**Fig. 1, Table 1**).

ADVERSE DRUG REACTIONS TO TOPICAL MEDICATIONS

With regard to the ADRs of the lower extremity, the initial evaluation should include a thorough work-up of common skin eruptions of this region, such as allergic contact dermatitis and stasis dermatitis, followed by the standard evaluation for an ADR. Topical drug contact dermatitis is common in this area of the body because of the frequent nature of application of various topical medications to manage chronic conditions such as stasis dermatitis and ulcerations, among other problems that are specific to the lower extremity.

Certain medications, such as topical antihistamines, most notably topical doxepin, sensitize more often when applied topically compared with when they are administered orally. Transdermal patches have become a more common route for medication delivery, and reports of sensitization have increased with nitroglycerin, hormones, nicotine, clonidine, lidocaine, scopolamine, and fentanyl delivered in this manner. Of the medications given via transdermal patches, clonidine induces the highest rate of allergic reactions.[5]

Patients with chronic leg ulcers are at much higher risk of developing contact dermatitis to various topical antibiotics, most notably neomycin and bacitracin. The clinical presentation of neomycin sensitivity of the lower extremity can be varied because chronic cutaneous changes have often developed. Early signs are pruritic, eczematous plaques but, with prolonged use, lichenified or hyperkeratotic papules and plaques may evolve. Similar findings may be found between the toes when this medication is erroneously used to treat dermatophytosis.[6] Bacitracin sensitivity may present similarly; however, contact urticaria, and even anaphylaxis, are reported more often with bacitracin than with any other antibiotic. For this reason, overuse of these medications is discouraged.[7]

Dermatophytosis of the lower legs, feet, and nails is common, and reactions to topical antifungal agents may occur. Allergic contact dermatitis to imidazole, with a

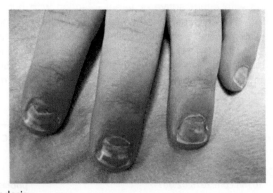

Fig. 1. Onychomadesis.

Table 1	
Adverse drug reactions in nails	
Affected Area	**Symptoms**
Matrix	Nail fragility
	Beau lines/onychomadesis
	True leukonychia
	Melanonychia
Nail bed	Onycholysis
	Photo-onycholysis
	Apparent leukonychia
	Dermal pigmentation
	Hemorrhagic onycholysis
Nail folds	Paronychia
	Pyogenic granuloma

high cross-reactivity rate to miconazole, clotrimazole, oxiconazole, and isoconazole may occur.

Stasis dermatitis is a cutaneous eruption associated with lower extremity swelling with an underlying vascular cause that initially produces cutaneous eczematous plaques that are often pruritic. As a result, topical corticosteroids are frequently used to manage the symptoms of inflammation and pruritus, and contact sensitization to these compounds may occur. Corticosteroids are separated into 4 structural classes, and classed class A, B, C, and D. Patch testing is the best tool for determining the causal agent.[8]

Nail changes typically occur with systemic agents; however, topical medications may induce nail changes. These changes are usually irritant or allergic contact dermatitis changes of the distal digit or dyschromia of the nail plate.[4]

ADVERSE DRUG REACTIONS TO SYSTEMIC AGENTS

Well-described ADRs to systemic agents include morbilliform exanthems; drug-induced hypersensitivity syndrome; and specific hypersensitivity syndromes to anticonvulsants, allopurinol, sulfonamides, minocycline, and dapsone that are well described and tend to involve many body areas beyond the lower extremities. In addition, bullous drug eruptions including toxic epidermal necrolysis and Stevens-Johnson syndrome involve multiple body areas, most notably the mucosa. These eruptions are more generalized and do not necessarily involve the lower extremities and are thus beyond the scope of this article. However, there are several ADRs to systemic agents that may specifically involve the lower extremities and/or nail apparatus that are covered in detail.

FIXED DRUG ERUPTIONS

Fixed drug eruptions (FDEs) are a common ADR. The reaction develops briskly; from 30 minutes to 8 hours from the time of ingestion of the drug to the development of skin findings, with an average of just 2 hours. FDEs recur at the same site with each reexposure of the drug. The clinical presentation of an FDE is typically a red patch that evolves into a targetoid patch that then may blister or erode. Larger plaques may occur, resembling cellulitis, especially when located on the distal lower extremity. The eroded plaque heals completely with appropriate wound care and withdrawal of the agent, but characteristically leaves postinflammatory hyperpigmentation.[9]

With continued ingestion of the offending drug, more lesions may develop on other body areas. Skin biopsy of the lesion reveals a characteristic pattern.

Drugs known to induce FDEs are usually drugs that are taken intermittently. NSAIDs, especially the pyrazolone derivatives, naproxen, oxicams, sulfonamides, trimethoprim, barbiturates, fluconazole, fluoroquinolones, tetracyclines, acetamino-phen, cetirizine, celecoxib, dextromethorphan, hydroxyzine, quinine, erythromycin, Chinese herbs, and lamotrigine are all high on the long list of medications reported to cause FDE.[10,11]

Although less common, FDEs may not result in postinflammatory hyperpigmenta-tion. This so-called nonpigmenting variant has 2 variants, 1 of which is limited to flex-ural or intertriginous areas, and the other that may occur on the lower extremities, known as the pseudocellulitis or scarlatiniform type. The latter type typically presents with large, tender, deeply erythematous plaques on the lower extremities that resolve completely without residual pigmentation over the course of 2 weeks. An identical eruption in the same location recurs on reingestion of the offending drug.[12]

MEDICATION-INDUCED LOWER LEG EDEMA

Lower leg edema occurs most often as a result of venous hypertension and subse-quent pooling of interstitial fluid secondary to venous valve incompetence. It charac-teristically occurs in both lower extremities, although not necessarily symmetrically. This condition can then lead to the acute phase of stasis dermatitis, with erythema, crusting, and pruritus, and ultimately to the chronic phase with hemosiderin hyperpig-mentation and subsequent lipodermatosclerosis.[13]

Several medications may cause lower extremity edema, and should be considered in any patient with new-onset lower extremity edema, with or without the associated changes of stasis dermatitis (**Table 2**).

ERYTHEMA NODOSUM CAUSED BY MEDICATIONS

Erythema nodosum is the most frequent variant of panniculitis, and characteristically causes the sudden onset of tender, erythematous, subcutaneous nodules on the ante-rior aspects of the distal lower extremities that eventually resolve without scarring. It may be associated with several disorders, such as infections and autoimmune syndromes, but medication-induced cases have been reported.[14] A large number of medications have been implicated as the cause for erythema nodosum, with the most frequent causal agents thought to be sulfonamides, bromides, and oral contra-ceptives. The situation becomes difficult when a patient is placed on antibiotics for an infection and subsequently develops erythema nodosum. In this circumstance, it can be difficult to determine whether the erythema nodosum is caused by the medication or the infection.[15]

MEDICATION-INDUCED PIGMENTATION OF THE SKIN

Drugs may induce pigmentation in the skin, either by postinflammatory hyperpigmen-tation or by the deposition of the drug in the skin. There are several drugs that cause pigmentation of the skin of the lower extremities and/or nails.

Minocycline induces several well-described forms of pigmentation, which may occur in combination within the same patient. Type I is a blue-black discoloration that appears in areas of previous inflammation, such as surgical scars or traumatic scars, and that may be located on the lower extremities. This type is not associated with the total or daily dose of exposure to the minocycline, although the incidence

Table 2
Medications associated with edema of the lower leg

	Drug Class	Medications
Alpha-adrenergic Antagonists	—	—
Antidepressants	Monoamine oxidase inhibitors	—
Antihypertensive medications	Calcium channel blockers	Benzothiazepines, dihydropyridines, phenylalkylamines
	β-Blockers	—
	Direct vasodilators	Diazoxide, hydralazine, minoxidil
	Clonidine	
	Methyldopa	
	Antisympathetic agents	Guanethidine, Reserpine
Antirheumatic agents	—	—
Chemotherapeutic agents	—	—
Endothelial receptor antagonists	—	Ambrisentan, Bosentan
Erythropoietic Agents	—	—
Hormones	Corticosteroids	—
	Estrogens/progesterones	
	Testosterone	
	Antibiotics	Levofloxacin
NSAIDs	—	Nonselective Cox-2 Inhibitors, phenylbutazone, selective Cox-2 inhibitors
Pregabalin	—	—
Thiazolidinediones	—	Pioglitazone, rosiglitazone, troglitazone

Abbreviation: Cox-2, cyclooxygenase-2.
Adapted from Hyman DA, Cohen PR. Stasis dermatitis as a complication of recurrent levofloxacin-associated bilateral leg edema. Dermatol Online J 2013;19(11):20399.

increases with increasing total dose. Type II is blue-black or blue-grey pigmentation on the anterior shins. The presentation resembles ecchymosis, but fades extremely slowly. Type III is the least common form, and is a muddy-brown hyperpigmentation that has a predilection for sun-exposed areas.[16]

Antimalarial agents chloroquine, hydroxychloroquine, and quinacrine all may cause a blue-black pigmentation, most often in the pretibial pattern of the lower extremity, similar to that induced by minocycline, but may also involve the nails. Quinidine may also cause this pattern of hyperpigmentation of the shins.

Chlorpromazine, thioridazine, imipramine, clomipramine, and amiodarone may all cause slate-grey hyperpigmentation in sun-exposed areas, which may include the tops of the feet or distal lower extremities.[17]

Chemotherapy agents cause dyspigmentation in characteristic patterns on the extremities. Doxorubicin and hydroxyurea cause hyperpigmentation of the nails and skin, most often in patients of African descent. Imatinib has reported to cause hyperpigmentation of the nails and skin, or localized depigmentation resembling vitiligo. Progression of vitiligo caused by imatinib has been reported in a patient. Given the acral predilection for vitiligo, awareness of this with regard to lower extremities is paramount.[18,19]

5-Fluorouracil (5-FU) has been reported to cause a characteristic supravenous hyperpigmented eruption in conjunction with bilateral mottling of the palms, and notable diffuse hyperpigmentation of the soles. Changing the peripheral venous route to a central line can improve this adverse drug reaction.[20]

Sunitinib may cause yellowing of the skin. Eruptive melanocytic nevi and lentigines with an acral predilection have been seen with sorafenib.[21]

MEDICATION-INDUCED PIGMENTATION OF THE NAILS

Pigmentation of the nails caused by medications can be of melanocytic or nonmelanocytic origin. When a drug activates the melanocytes of the nail matrix, the melanocytes may only be partially activated, and as such only a group of matrix melanocytes are activated to produce pigment, and a longitudinal pigmented band known as melanonychia striata results. If there is diffuse activation of most or all of the melanocytes in the affected matrix, there will be pigmentation of the entire nail plate. Less commonly, this drug-induced melanocyte activation results in the appearance of pigmented transverse bands that are parallel to the lunula, alternating with bands of normal color, indicating intermittent melanin production. Drug-induced melanonychia typically arises in the distal matrix.[4,22]

Nail pigmentation caused by melanocyte activation leading to melanin deposition in the nail plate is a frequent side effect of chemotherapeutic agents doxorubicin, bleomycin, cyclophosphamide, daunorubicin, dacarbazine, 5-FU, methotrexate, and hydroxyurea. Transverse pigmented bands caused by intermittent melanin production can be seen with psoralen with ultraviolet A, infliximab, and zidovudine, as well as the synthetic Melanotan injections.[4]

Nonmelanocytic pigmentation caused by medications has a different pathogenesis. Certain medications are deposited in the nail matrix as a way of eliminating the drug. The deposition of the drug within the plate causes the plate to appear brown, specifically in patients treated with clofazimine. Other causes of nonmelanocytic pigmentation include deposition of pigments in the dermis of the periungual region. In this case, the pigmentation is not within the plate, and thus does not move forward with nail growth, and is often associated with pigmentation of the skin elsewhere. Minocycline has been reported to cause nails to appear a blue-grey color, but typically spares the lunula.[22]

A blue, brown, or grey pigmentation that does not move distally with growth can be seen in patients treated with long-term antimalarial therapy, including amodiaquine; chloroquine; mepacrine; quinacrine; or, most rarely, hydroxychloroquine.[23]

Zidovudine causes a characteristic blue or brown hyperpigmentation of the nails, with blue lunulae and/or dark brown nail plates. This condition may or may not be accompanied by diffuse hyperpigmentation of the skin.[24]

SKIN NECROSIS CAUSED BY ANTICOAGULANTS

Although both warfarin and heparin may cause cutaneous necrosis, warfarin-induced skin necrosis (WISN) seems to occur most frequently in the lower extremities. WISN occurs within several days of initiating therapy, with painful red plaques that evolve into large bullae. Although lesions tend to occur in areas abundant in subcutaneous fat, a variant may be seen in the lower extremity in patients with deep venous thrombosis (DVT). The necrosis occurs in the limb with the DVT. WISN occurs most often in patients with cancer.

Heparin induces necrosis in a widespread pattern that may or may not involve the lower extremity. Unfractionated heparin is more likely to cause cutaneous necrosis than fractionated low-molecular-weight heparin.[25–27]

ADVERSE DRUG REACTIONS TO CHEMOTHERAPEUTIC AGENTS

Chemotherapeutic agents cause ADRs via a multitude of mechanisms. These reactions may be related to toxicity directly to a skin appendage, such as the sweat gland, or to another organ system that results in skin changes, such as purpura caused by thrombocytopenia. In addition, these agents may induce classic immunologic drug reactions. There are several chemotherapy-induced ADRs that specifically affect the lower extremity.

CHEMOTHERAPY-INDUCED ACRAL ERYTHEMA

Chemotherapy-induced acral erythema, also known as palmoplantar erythrodysesthesia syndrome or hand-foot syndrome, is a common syndrome that occurs most frequently from administration of doxorubicin, cytosine arabinoside, and 5-FU but also has been reported to occur with docetaxel, capecitabine, and high-dose liposomal doxorubicin and daunorubicin.[28,29]

The initial clinical presentation often begins with dysesthesia of the palms and soles, followed a few days later with painful and symmetric erythema and edema of the volar surface of the digits. The eruption may extend to the dorsal surface of the hands and feet. The eruption progresses over the following days to a dusky hue, then blisters and desquamates, followed by reepithelialization. The desquamation is the most notable and characteristic part of this syndrome. Full-thickness ischemic necrosis may occur in the areas of blistering/desquamation.

The pathogenesis is thought to be caused by a direct toxic effect of the chemotherapeutic agents on the skin via the sweat glands. The sweat glands concentrate the agent, and these glands deliver the chemotherapy onto the surface of the skin. The high concentration of sweat glands on the palms and soles explains the pattern of this syndrome.

Cooling of the hands and feet during chemotherapy administration in order to decrease the concentration of the agents in these areas and/or modification of the dose schedule may decrease the severity of the reaction.[28,29]

CHEMOTHERAPY-INDUCED DERMATOLOGIC CHANGES INVOLVING THE LOWER EXTREMITY CAUSED BY VARIOUS CHEMOTHERAPY AGENTS

For patients undergoing chemotherapy with coexisting lymphedema of the lower extremities, it is important to consider that gemcitabine, an antimetabolite, has been reported to induce pseudocellulitis in areas of preexisting lymphedema. It is thought that the areas of lymphedema may increase the concentration of gemcitabine and reduce its rate of metabolism.[30]

Multikinase inhibitors, such as sorafenib and sunitinib, induce a condition that resembles hand-foot syndrome, known as hand-foot skin reaction (HFSR). Patients present similarly, initially with acral dysesthesia and pain, but it is typically less severe and without the associated edema. HFSR also induces pronounced hyperkeratotic plaques over areas of friction, such as the heels and ankles with regard to the lower extremities. Nail changes may also occur, and include painful subungual hemorrhages 2 to 4 weeks after the start of treatment. HFSR is dose dependent, and worsens with the addition of another multikinase inhibitor to the regimen.

Multikinase inhibitors may cause other skin reactions. Imatinib may cause exacerbation of psoriasis, acral psoriasiform hyperkeratosis, or lichenoid drug eruption with palmoplantar hyperkeratosis; bevacizumab may interfere with wound healing, and both sorafenib and nilotinib may cause the rapid eruptive keratoacanthomas or squamous cell carcinomas.[31,32]

B-Raf proto-oncogene inhibitors, including vemurafenib and dabrafenib, have also been associated with eruptive keratoacanthomas and squamous cell carcinomas. In addition, they may cause erythematous, granulomatous papules that involve the distal lower extremities. These papules resolve with potent topical steroids without withdrawal of therapy.[33]

Patients treated with docetaxel or paclitaxel may develop a sclerodermalike reaction that may occur after 1 or several treatments with these taxanes. Patients acutely develop diffuse, infiltrative edema of the extremities and head. The lower extremities become sclerotic and painful over the following months. Flexion contractures of the palms, soles, and digits may occur. Most cases resolve with discontinuation of therapy. A similar reaction has been reported with pemetrexed.[19,34]

CHEMOTHERAPY-INDUCED NAIL CHANGES

Nail toxicity is common during chemotherapy, and is thought to occur in up to 44% of patients who have received taxanes. Chemotherapy-induced nail changes caused by toxicity of the nail matrix range from thinning and fragility of the nail, to disruption or slowing of the nail matrix causing either Beau lines or complete onychomadesis, or proximal nail shedding. Onychomadesis is an extreme degree of Beau lines, with more extensive slowing or cessation of nail matrix activity. Onychomadesis is most common in patients treated with high-dose chemotherapy, but has been reported with carbamazepine, lithium carbonate, cephaloridine, and cloxacillin.[4]

Chemotherapy-induced nail changes caused by toxic damage of the keratinocytes of the nail bed include onycholysis, or separation of the nail plate from the nail bed, causing a new space between the bed and plate that appears white. Onycholysis caused by medications may be the result of damage to the nail bed epithelium, causing poor adhesion, or, in more extreme cases, the drug causes total destruction of the nail bed epithelium and the formation of a hemorrhagic blister. This blister, caused by nail bed epithelium destruction, is extremely painful, and is often associated with blistering on the soles of the feet.

Painful, hemorrhagic onycholysis may occur with the use of taxanes (docetaxel, paclitaxel) and doxorubicin (**Fig. 2**). These nail changes are intensely painful, and the onycholysis is often dose related. Although it regresses spontaneously after discontinuation of the offending agent, healing may take months. Patients often experience relief

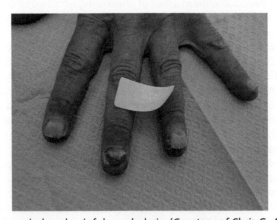

Fig. 2. Chemotherapy-induced painful onycholysis. (*Courtesy of* Chris G. Adigun, MD.)

in their symptoms when the nail finally falls off, because the pain is frequently caused by the pressure of the nail plate on the fragile and sensitive nail bed.[19]

Chemotherapy-induced nail changes caused by toxicity and damage to the proximal and lateral nail folds can lead to paronychia and pyogenic granulomas. The medications cause the nail folds to become intensely swollen and painful. Acute paronychia caused by toxic damage to the proximal nail fold is commonly caused by taxanes but also occurs with epidermal growth factor receptor (EGFR) inhibitors such as cetuximab and gefitinib.[22]

Drug-induced pyogenic granulomas (PGs) frequently involve the nail unit, usually both fingers and toes, although toes are more commonly affected because the toenails are vulnerable to chronic friction from shoes and carrying body weight. EGFR inhibitors, including erlotinib, lapatinib, cetuximab, and panitumumab, cause paronychia and PG formation in up to 60% of patients.[35] It is dose dependent. Capecitabine, a 5-FU prodrug, may also cause periungual PGs.

ADVERSE REACTIONS TO IMMUNOSUPPRESSIVE OR IMMUNOMODULATORY AGENTS

The tumor necrosis factor (TNF) inhibitors are used for various autoimmune conditions, including rheumatoid arthritis and psoriasis. These biologic medications are associated with several adverse reactions that may affect the lower extremities. These reactions include palmoplantar pustulosis, pustular folliculitis, worsening of psoriasis, neutrophilic eccrine hidradenitis, and vasculitis. This paradoxic development of psoriasis while on these antipsoriatic therapies has been reported with the 3 most common TNF inhibitors: infliximab, etanercept, and adalimumab. The psoriasis eruption may occur within weeks to years of initiation of therapy, with the palmoplantar pustulosis morphologic variant being the most common, responsible for 40% of cases. Most patients have improvement or resolution with discontinuation of therapy.[36,37]

Methotrexate is an antimitotic agent that has been the mainstay of treatment of various autoimmune conditions, including rheumatoid arthritis and psoriasis. Although methotrexate has numerous potential side effects, one that is notable to affect the lower extremities is its ability to cause cutaneous ulceration. These ulcers can be widespread, but tend to concentrate on the extremities, and are often associated with bone marrow suppression. Withdrawal of the methotrexate and supportive care should lead to complete resolution of the ulcers.[38]

Various nail changes have been reported with immunosuppressive agents, including melanocytic pigmentation from infliximab and painful hemorrhagic onycholysis from sirolimus and rituximab.[4]

OTHER NAIL CHANGES CAUSED BY MEDICATIONS

Photo-onycholysis is the separation of the nail plate from the nail bed as a result of either an allergic or toxic effect of the drug that is caused by or activated by ultraviolet radiation. Although more common on the fingers, it can theoretically happen on the toes in an individual taking the offending agent and exposing the feet and toes to ultraviolet radiation.[39] The drugs that most commonly cause this phenomenon are tetracyclines and psoralens. This condition may occur from either natural sources of ultraviolet light such as the sun, or from artificial ultraviolet lamps (**Box 1**).

Systemic and topical retinoids both can cause nail fragility, paronychia, and periungual PGs. The increased fragility of the nail is thought to contribute to the high incidence of ingrown toenails and periungual PGs. The fragile nail plate splits and breaks easily, forming a nail spicule that easily penetrates the lateral nail fold. This

| **Box 1** |
| **Drugs reported to cause photo-onycholysis** |
| Tetracyclines |
| Psoralens |
| Fluoroquinolones |
| Quinine |
| Clorazepate dipotassium |
| Indapamide |
| Benoxaprofen |
| Olanzapine and aripiprazole |
| Aminolevulanic acid |
| Griseofulvin |

spicula, together with the retinoid-induced increased propensity to form granulation tissue, leads to the formation of ingrown toenails and PGs in these patients.[4]

REFERENCES

1. Dodiuk-Gad RP, Laws PM, Shear NH. Epidemiology of severe drug hypersensitivity. Semin Cutan Med Surg 2014;33(1):2–9.
2. de la Torre C, Suh Oh HJ. Advances in the diagnosis of drug eruptions. Actas Dermosifiliogr 2013;104(9):782–8.
3. Harp JL, Kinnebrew MA, Shinkai K. Severe cutaneous adverse reactions: impact of immunology, genetics, and pharmacology. Semin Cutan Med Surg 2014;33(1):17–27.
4. Piraccini BM, Alessandrini A. Drug-related nail disease. Clin Dermatol 2013;31(5):618–26.
5. Musel AL, Warshaw EM. Cutaneous reactions to transdermal therapeutic systems. Dermatitis 2006;17(3):109–22.
6. Jean SE, Moreau L. Contact dermatitis in leg ulcer patients. J Cutan Med Surg 2009;13(Suppl 1):S38–41.
7. Cronin H, Mowad C. Anaphylactic reaction to bacitracin ointment. Cutis 2009;83(3):127–9.
8. Isaksson M. Systemic contact allergy to corticosteroids revisited. Contact Dermatitis 2007;57(6):386–8.
9. Jang KA, Choi JH, Sung KS, et al. Idiopathic eruptive macular pigmentation: report of 10 cases. J Am Acad Dermatol 2001;44(2 Suppl):351–3.
10. Hiware S, Shrivastava M, Mishra D, et al. Evaluation of cutaneous drug reactions in patients visiting out patient departments of Indira Gandhi Government Medical College and Hospital (IGGMC and H), Nagpur. Indian J Dermatol 2013;58(1):18–21.
11. Shrivastava MP, Chaudhari HV, Dakhale GN, et al. Adverse drug reactions related to the use of non-steroidal anti-inflammatory drugs: results of spontaneous reporting from central India. J Indian Med Assoc 2013;111(2):99–102, 106.
12. Winnicki M, Shear NH. A systematic approach to systemic contact dermatitis and symmetric drug-related intertriginous and flexural exanthema (SDRIFE): a closer

look at these conditions and an approach to intertriginous eruptions. Am J Clin Dermatol 2011;12(3):171–80.

13. Hyman DA, Cohen PR. Stasis dermatitis as a complication of recurrent levofloxacin-associated bilateral leg edema. Dermatol Online J 2013;19(11): 20399.

14. Gheith O, Al-Otaibi T, Tawab KA, et al. Erythema nodosum in renal transplant recipients: multiple cases and review of literature. Transpl Infect Dis 2010;12(2): 164–8.

15. Requena L, Yus ES. Erythema nodosum. Dermatol Clin 2008;26(4):425–38.

16. Geria AN, Tajirian AL, Kihiczak G, et al. Minocycline-induced skin pigmentation: an update. Acta Dermatovenerol Croat 2009;17(2):123–6.

17. Grimes P, Nordlund JJ, Pandya AG, et al. Increasing our understanding of pigmentary disorders. J Am Acad Dermatol 2006;54(5 Suppl 2):S255–61.

18. Reyes-Habito CM, Roh EK. Cutaneous reactions to chemotherapeutic drugs and targeted therapy for cancer: part II. Targeted therapy. J Am Acad Dermatol 2014; 71(2):217.e1–11 [quiz: 227–8].

19. Reyes-Habito CM, Roh EK. Cutaneous reactions to chemotherapeutic drugs and targeted therapies for cancer: part I. Conventional chemotherapeutic drugs. J Am Acad Dermatol 2014;71(2):203.e1–12 [quiz: 215–6].

20. Suvirya S, Agrawal A, Parihar A. 5-Fluorouracil-induced bilateral persistent serpentine supravenous hyperpigmented eruption, bilateral mottling of palms and diffuse hyperpigmentation of soles. BMJ Case Rep 2014;2014:1–3.

21. Uhlenhake EE, Watson AC, Aronson P. Sorafenib induced eruptive melanocytic lesions. Dermatol Online J 2013;19(5):18184.

22. Zaiac MN, Walker A. Nail abnormalities associated with systemic pathologies. Clin Dermatol 2013;31(5):627–49.

23. Kalabalikis D, Patsatsi A, Trakatelli MG, et al. Hyperpigmented forearms and nail: a quiz. Acta Derm Venereol 2010;90(6):657–9.

24. Piraccini BM, Tosti A. Drug-induced nail disorders: incidence, management and prognosis. Drug Saf 1999;21(3):187–201.

25. Choudhry S, Fishman PM, Hernandez C. Heparin-induced bullous hemorrhagic dermatosis. Cutis 2013;91(2):93–8.

26. Mungalsingh CR, Bomford J, Nayagam J, et al. Warfarin-induced skin necrosis. Clin Med (Lond) 2012;12(1):90–1.

27. Tassava T, Warkentin TE. Non-injection-site necrotic skin lesions complicating postoperative heparin thromboprophylaxis. Am J Hematol 2015;90(8):747–50.

28. Nakano K, Komatsu K, Kubo T, et al. Hand-foot skin reaction is associated with the clinical outcome in patients with metastatic renal cell carcinoma treated with sorafenib. Jpn J Clin Oncol 2013;43(10):1023–9.

29. Nardone B, Hensley JR, Kulik L, et al. The effect of hand-foot skin reaction associated with the multikinase inhibitors sorafenib and sunitinib on health-related quality of life. J Drugs Dermatol 2012;11(11):e61–5.

30. Curtis S, Hong S, Gucalp R, et al. Gemcitabine-induced pseudocellulitis in a patient with recurrent lymphedema: a case report and review of the current literature. Am J Ther 2016;23(1):e321–3.

31. Kuraishi N, Nagai Y, Hasegawa M, et al. Lichenoid drug eruption with palmoplantar hyperkeratosis due to imatinib mesylate: a case report and a review of the literature. Acta Derm Venereol 2010;90(1):73–6.

32. Peters P, Rabbolini D, Sinnya S, et al. Multiple squamous cell carcinomas following introduction of nilotinib. Clin Exp Dermatol 2014;39(7):791–4.

33. Park JJ, Hawryluk EB, Tahan SR, et al. Cutaneous granulomatous eruption and successful response to potent topical steroids in patients undergoing targeted BRAF inhibitor treatment for metastatic melanoma. JAMA Dermatol 2014; 150(3):307–11.

34. Corbaux C, Marie J, Meraud JP, et al. Pemetrexed-induced scleroderma-like changes in the lower legs. Ann Dermatol Venereol 2015;142(2):115–20.

35. Piraccini BM, Bellavista S, Misciali C, et al. Periungual and subungual pyogenic granuloma. Br J Dermatol 2010;163(5):941–53.

36. Hawryluk EB, Linskey KR, Duncan LM, et al. Broad range of adverse cutaneous eruptions in patients on TNF-alpha antagonists. J Cutan Pathol 2012;39(5): 481–92.

37. Peluso R, Cafaro G, Di Minno A, et al. Side effects of TNF-α blockers in patients with psoriatic arthritis: evidences from literature studies. Clin Rheumatol 2013; 32(6):743–53.

38. Kurian A, Haber R. Methotrexate-induced cutaneous ulcers in a nonpsoriatic patient: case report and review of the literature. J Cutan Med Surg 2011;15(5): 275–9.

39. Badri T, Ben Tekaya N, Cherif F, et al. Photo-onycholysis: two cases induced by doxycycline. Acta Dermatovenerol Alp Pannonica Adriat 2004;13(4):135–6.

Melanoma of the Foot

Ivan Bristow, PhD, FFPM RCPS (Glasg)[a],*, Chris Bower, MB ChB, FRCP[b]

KEYWORDS

- Skin • Cancer • Melanoma • Acral • Foot • Nail

KEY POINTS

- Melanoma of the foot has many unique characteristics compared with cutaneous melanoma elsewhere in terms of its presentation and prognosis.
- Melanoma of the foot is frequently delayed in its presentation and diagnosis because of its highly variable appearance on the plantar surface and within the nail unit.
- To assist practitioners in earlier recognition the CUBED (colored, uncertain diagnosis, bleeding, enlargement, delay) acronym can help to increase awareness of a possible foot melanoma diagnosis. In addition, the dermatoscope is a useful clinical tool that can improve clinical assessment of suspicious lesions.
- New drug therapies targeting known melanoma mutations are showing promise in the treatment of melanoma, extending survival times for patients with the disease.

INTRODUCTION

The increase in incidence of cutaneous malignant melanoma worldwide continues to be of concern with around 132,000 new cases occurring globally every year.[1] Despite these increases, some data suggest that mortality from the disease is levelling, probably because of an increase in public awareness and earlier diagnosis of the disease.[2] However, melanoma that arises on the foot represents a subset of the disease, compared with cutaneous melanoma (CM) elsewhere, that runs counter to these observed improvements. Foot melanoma has its own unique peculiarities and clinically may present a greater diagnostic challenge because lesions often are presented and diagnosed late, adversely affecting outcomes. Recent research has shown dermoscopy to improve recognition of early lesions but, despite promising advances in treatment of established disease, excision remains the mainstay of therapy.

TYPES OF MELANOMA

A melanoma is a malignant tumor arising from the melanocyte. The tumor can arise on any area of the skin, and up to half occur in preexisting melanocytic nevi.[3] Melanoma

Disclosure: The authors have nothing to disclose.
[a] Faculty of Health Sciences, University of Southampton, Southampton SO17 1BJ, UK;
[b] Department of Dermatology, Royal Devon and Exeter NHS Foundation Trust, Gladstone Road, Exeter EX1 2ED, UK
* Corresponding author.
E-mail address: i.bristow@soton.ac.uk

can be categorized into subtypes based on histology and pathologic characteristics. Lesions arising on the foot and hands, particularly the palms, soles, or within the nails, are often termed acral or volar melanomas; a reference to anatomic location rather than their subtype. Although not all melanomas are classifiable, the main subtypes of melanoma that may arise on the skin are:

- Superficial spreading melanoma (SSM) (**Fig. 1**)
- Lentigo maligna melanoma (LMM)
- Nodular melanoma (NM) (**Fig. 2**)
- Acral lentiginous melanoma (ALM) (**Fig. 3**)

Across the whole body surface, SSM accounts for around 65% of all melanomas, whereas LLM accounts for 27%, NM 7%, and ALM just 1%.[4] However, on the foot, the ALM subtype predominates, being responsible for around 60% of all foot melanoma, with SSM and NM accounting for 30% and 9% respectively.[5] Other investigators have concluded similar proportions, with the ALM subtypes being the most prevalent lesion type,[6,7] and with LMM being rarely found in areas other than the head and neck.

AMELANOTIC MELANOMA

Within each of the main subtypes, a proportion of lesions may be categorized as amelanotic (or hypopigmented), in which, instead of being the usual dark brown/black color, lesions may be devoid of pigment, appearing lighter in color (ie, pink or red) (**Fig. 4**). Across the whole body, less than 8% of melanoma are classified as amelanotic[8]; however, within the specific subtypes hypomelanotic or amelanotic lesions may represent much higher percentages. Around 40% of NM and ALM have been shown to have reduced or no pigment within them,[9] with amelanotic lesions being seen more frequently in areas such as the palms and soles.[10]

NAIL MELANOMA

Nail melanoma is not specifically a histologic subtype of melanoma but merely refers to lesions arising from within the nail unit (**Fig. 5**). Most of these lesions are ALM or NM. Melanoma arising in the nail unit is rare and accounts for less than 2% of all melanoma cases.[11] Because many lesions are nail unit located ALM, this type of melanoma occurs equally in all races.

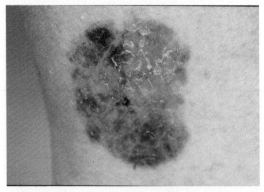

Fig. 1. SSM. A type that spreads radially before gradually becoming vertically invasive. On the foot, most melanomas of this subtype are found on the dorsum.

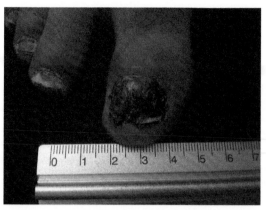

Fig. 2. NM (affecting the nail). A more aggressive melanoma than the SSM because it may rapidly become vertically invasive. The lesion is most common in older patients. (*From* Bristow I, Dalton A. A late diagnosis of nail melanoma arising in the hallux. Podiatry Now 2013;16(4):21–3.)

Figs. 1–5 show the main variants of melanoma arising on the foot.[10]

HOW COMMON IS MELANOMA ON THE FOOT?

The proportion of melanomas that occur on the foot is difficult to accurately ascertain because epidemiologic studies have rarely categorized lesions on the foot exclusively, tending to amalgamate them with lesions of the hand or with the lower extremity, making accurate estimates difficult. One recent study of 1542 melanomas identified 6.6% of lesions as arising on the foot, with a slight female preponderance, which has been observed in other studies.[12] However, wide variation of this figure can be seen among different ethnic groups.

Nonwhite races, despite having a have a much lower rate of the disease generally, are more likely to develop lesions in acral locations such as the palmar, plantar surfaces and nail bed.[13] For example, Jimbow and colleagues[14] reported that 40% of melanomas occurring in their Japanese cohort of patients were in acral locations, with 80% of these lesions being diagnosed as ALM. The ALM is the most frequently observed type of the disease in nonwhite populations.[15] Although melanoma can arise at virtually any age, it is rare before adulthood, increasing in incidence with

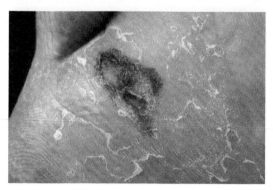

Fig. 3. ALM. The rarer subtype of the disease, but is most common on the foot, particularly on the soles and in the nail unit. This subtype occurs at the same rate in all races/skin types.

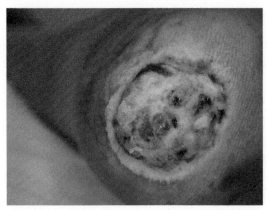

Fig. 4. Amelanotic melanoma. Several melanomas may lack pigment and are classed as amelanotic. Amelanotic lesions are more frequent in acral areas such as the foot and are diagnostically more challenging.

age, with most melanomas on the foot arising between the sixth and eighth decades of life.[7]

CAUSE

Intermittent and chronic sun exposure along with a history of sunburns is the major factor that is associated the development of cutaneous malignant melanoma. However, lesions arising in areas that are seldom exposed to the sun, such as the nail unit and soles of the feet, bring into question the true cause for lesions in these areas; additional factors may contribute. For example, the nail unit has a small skin surface area but research has shown that melanoma density is 9 times the expected average for an area of this size.[16] In addition, much of the nail unit is shielded by the nail plate, which at a thickness of greater than 0.5 mm is a shield to virtually all ultraviolet B radiation reaching the nail bed.[17] Moreover, a recent study has highlighted how, despite increases in melanoma generally having occurred over the last few years, rates of melanoma on the foot have remained fairly constant.[18]

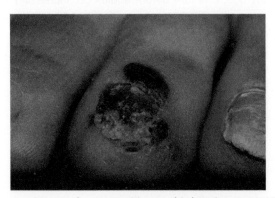

Fig. 5. Nail melanoma. Most melanomas arising at this location are ALM but occasionally NM. Lesions may arise initially as a longitudinal melanonychia or as alterations in nail plate.

The role of trauma and the development of melanoma has been much debated but still remains unresolved. By virtue of their location, the feet are likely to be subjected to more physical trauma than other areas of the body, which has bolstered the traumatic cause theory. Although patients frequently report injuries as a possible cause of their melanomas, few scientific studies have objectively substantiated these claims. It has been suggested that in many cases a traumatic event to the affected area only serves to focus the patient's attention to a previously existing lesion.[19]

Despite the lack of sun exposure to many areas of the foot, resemblance to melanoma elsewhere on the body has been shown. In a case-control study of white patients with palmar and plantar melanomas versus patients without melanoma, it was shown that patients with foot melanoma had a higher sun exposure level, higher total body mole count, and a greater history of sunburn.[20] The investigators suggest that, despite lack of sun exposure to the plantar surface, total sun exposure may positively affect the development of plantar lesions. The presence of preexisting plantar lesions was also found to be a risk factor. Higher levels of junctional and compound nevi in less sun-exposed sites, like the soles, have been suggested as an explanation for the occurrence of melanoma in these areas.[21] Exposure to agricultural and industrial chemicals has also been explored as a possible explanation, with an increased risk being observed in 1 systematic review.[22]

CLINICAL PRESENTATION OF MELANOMA ON THE FOOT

Timely diagnosis of melanoma relies on prompt presentation by patients to their health care professionals, which permits recognition and diagnosis by the treating clinician. Delays in patient presentation have been recognized as an issue. Consequently, patients may present with more advanced melanoma, adding to a poorer prognosis.

Thorough assessment of any potential skin cancer by a treating physician is a key stage in diagnosis; however, foot melanoma in particular frequently present challenges, resulting in diagnostic delay. Initial misdiagnosis rates for melanoma generally have been estimated at around 18%,[23] but figures for lesions arising on the foot have been shown to be much higher (25%–36%[24,25]) with the ALM subtype and nail melanoma offering the greatest diagnostic challenge.[26] Reasons for this are under-researched but, with a highly variable clinical appearance, it can resemble many common podiatric disorders, particularly when it is lacking in pigment. The literature contains many published case reports documenting melanoma misdiagnosed as more common skin conditions (**Box 1**).

The ABCDE (asymmetry, border, color, diameter, evolving) acronym has been used by the public and physicians in establishing suspicion of melanoma since 1985[27] (**Table 1**), but its utility in the diagnosis of smaller and amelanotic lesions, and those arising on the foot, has been questioned.[4,24] Recognizing the issues around delayed diagnosis and misdiagnosis, a new acronym, CUBED (colored, uncertain diagnosis, bleeding, enlargement, delay), has been proposed[10] (**Table 2**). Any lesion scoring 2 or more should be referred or considered for a biopsy.

More recently, in dermatology, the use of dermoscopy as part of the lesion assessment process has become mainstream.[28] The dermatoscope is a handheld device that offers magnification of the lesions (10×) and is used with gel or an oil-based medium or using polarized light, which allows visualization of structures not normally visible to the naked eye (**Fig. 6**). With training, use of the device has been shown to be more predictive in recognizing the potential signs of melanoma than the naked

---

Box 1
Reported misdiagnoses for melanoma on the foot

Ingrowing toe nail

Foot ulcer

Wart/verrucae

Tinea pedis/onychomycosis

Bruising

Foreign body

Subungual hematoma

Pyogenic granuloma

Poroma

Hyperkeratosis (corns/callus)

Necrosis

Paronychia

Ganglion

---

eye.[29] Consequently, it allows earlier recognition of melanoma before it becomes advanced and reduces the excision rates for benign lesions. Moreover, having such a device increases clinicians' awareness of the need for vigilant assessment of pigmented lesions.[30]

PRESENTATION OF MELANOMA OF THE NAIL UNIT

Nail melanomas typically present late and subsequently hold a poorer prognosis. Their variable appearance and rarity can make them a significant diagnostic challenge. Typically, lesions present in 2 ways. First, as a longitudinal melanonychia stripe that eventually alters normal nail anatomy; or, second, as an amelanotic tumor that gives rise to some nail plate disruption. Subungual bleeding is a common clinical condition that can give rise to diagnostic uncertainty. A good history and careful short-term observation can offer clues to discern possible causes; a subungual brown

Table 1
The ABCDE mnemonic

Letter	Meaning	Description
A	Asymmetry	One half of the lesion is not like the other half
B	Border	An irregular, scalloped, or poorly defined border
C	Color	Variegation of the colors
D	Diameter	Melanomas are usually larger than 6 mm but can be smaller
E	Evolving	A mole or lesion that is changing in size, shape, or color

Data from Friedman RJ, Rigel DS, Kopf AW. Early detection of malignant melanoma: the role of physician examination and self-examination of the skin. CA Cancer J Clin 1985;35(3):130–51; and Abbasi NR, Shaw HM, Rigel DS, et al. Early diagnosis of cutaneous melanoma: revisiting the ABCD criteria. JAMA 2004;292(22):2771–6.

Table 2	
The CUBED acronym	
C	Colored lesions of which any part is not skin color
U	Uncertain diagnosis. Any lesion that does not have a definite diagnosis
B	Bleeding lesions on the foot or under the nail, whether the bleeding is direct bleeding or oozing of fluid. This criterion includes chronic granulation tissue
E	Enlargement or deterioration of a lesion or ulcer despite therapy
D	Delay in healing of any lesion beyond 2 months

Consider undertaking a biopsy or specialist referral if any 2 or more criteria apply.
Adapted from Bristow IR, de Berker DA, Acland KM, et al. Clinical guidelines for the recognition of melanoma of the foot and nail unit. J Foot Ankle Res 2010;3:25.

discoloration that clears proximally with time is almost certainly a hematoma. Also, it is important to remember that functioning melanocytes are almost always exclusively found in the matrix and nail folds, so a longitudinal stripe that arises half way up in the nail bed is very unlikely to be a melanoma. **Table 3** highlights the characteristics that may help distinguish subungual bleeding from melanonychia.

Levit and colleagues[31] produced an ABCDE acronym to help in early recognition of nail melanoma, summarized in **Box 2**.

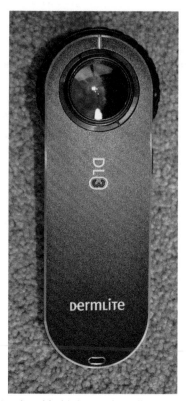

Fig. 6. The dermatoscope is a hand-held device that allows visualization of skin structures not normally observed by the naked eye. (*Courtesy of* 3Gen Inc, San Juan Capistrano, CA, with permission.)

Table 3
Features of longitudinal melanonychia compared with those of subungual bleeding; all features are generally true, but there can be individual exceptions

Melanonychia	Subungual Bleeding
The duration of history is 3–6 mo up to 20 y or more	The duration of history is rarely more than 6 mo and is typically shorter
A history of trauma is common	A history of trauma or precipitating activity is common
Lateral margins within the nail are mainly straight and longitudinally oriented	Lateral margins may be irregular
Where margins merge with the nail fold, pigment may spread onto nail fold (Hutchinson sign)	Pigment rarely extends from beneath the nail plate
There are rarely any detectable transverse features	There may be a proximal transverse groove and/or transverse white mark within the nail
In the absence of clinical tumor, nail plate pigmentation is in continuity with a single zone	Hemorrhage may be broken up into several zones
Dermoscopy reveals • Continuous pigment between proximal nail fold and distal free edge • In the transverse axis, pigment may vary, whereas in the longitudinal axis it remains largely constant • There may be longitudinal flecks of darker pigment within the background pigment of the nail • Pigment is mainly brown-black	Dermoscopy reveals • Pigment may not be continuous in the longitudinal axis, with clear nail at either the proximal or distal margin • Pigment may vary in any axis • Droplets of blood may be seen separated from the main zone of pigmentation • Blood may be seen as a discrete layer of material on the lower aspect of the nail plate at the free margin • Pigment may be purple-black, with increasing red hues at margins. It is rarely brown

Adapted from Bristow IR, de Berker DA, Acland KM, et al. Clinical guidelines for the recognition of melanoma of the foot and nail unit. J Foot Ankle Res 2010;3:25.

Box 2
The ABCDE of nail melanoma

A. Age range 20 to 90 years, peak fifth to seventh decades.

B. Band (nail band): pigment (brown-black). Breadth greater than 3 mm. Border (irregular/blurred).

C. Change: rapid increase in size/growth rate of nail band. Lack of change: failure of nail dystrophy to improve despite adequate treatment.

D. Digit involved (thumb > hallux > index finger > single digit > multiple digits).

E. Extension: extension of pigment to involve proximal or lateral nail fold (Hutchinson sign) or free edge of nail plate.

F. Family or personal history of previous melanoma or dysplastic nevus.

From Levit EK, Kagen MH, Scher RK, et al. The ABC rule for clinical detection of subungual melanoma. J Am Acad Dermatol 2000;42(2 Pt 1):271; with permission.

DERMOSCOPY

Dermoscopy in assessment of pigmented lesions on the feet has been found to be useful. The unique properties of thickened, weight-bearing plantar skin give rise to specific dermatoscopic patterns in benign and malignant melanomas. On the skin, close examination with the dermatoscope has shown that benign lesions have concentrated pigment patterns in the narrow furrows of the natural dermatoglyphics, which have been termed the parallel furrow pattern (**Fig. 7**). However, in malignant melanoma, pigmentation is frequently accentuated on the wider ridges of the dermatoglyphics along with lesion asymmetry and color variegation[32] (**Fig. 8**).

Dermoscopy has also been used as a technique for differentiating the various causes of melanonychia within the nail, including melanoma. Although currently untested formally, the technique has been shown to help inform clinicians' decisions on whether a nail biopsy is appropriate.[33]

DIAGNOSIS AND STAGING OF MELANOMA

A diagnosis of melanoma is made following histologic analysis and interpretation of the report on the excised lesion. In order to assess the extent of the disease, staging is an important step to determine the optimum treatment strategy and establish a prognosis. Melanoma staging (**Table 4**) is based on the following tumor characteristics: thickness of the tumor (Breslow thickness); the appearance of microscopic ulceration on the surface of a tumor, and the mitotic rate of cells within the tumor. Staging is also based on presence and type of any nodal and distant metastases.[34]

Patients with melanoma arising on the foot are clinically examined, with palpation of relevant lymph nodes in the groin of the affected limb. Any suspicious swelling is then be investigated further, usually with ultrasonography and needle biopsy. However, nodal metastases may be nondetectable with clinical examination.

For patients with melanoma considered to be at higher risk of lymph node metastasis, sentinel lymph node biopsy (SLNB) can be considered. This technique is performed under general anesthetic at the time of wide local excision. A mildly radioactive dye is injected into the skin at the site of the previously excised melanoma. Dye is then tracked to the first group of lymph nodes, possibly aided by the use of a radioactivity scanner. One or more of these nodes (the sentinel nodes) are then excised and examined histologically. The presence of melanoma in a sentinel node usually indicates the need for excision of all the regional lymph nodes from that site (lymphadenectomy).

SLNB is a technique to accurately stage melanomas. However, it is not a treatment of melanoma. Lymphadenectomy can reduce the risk of regional melanoma

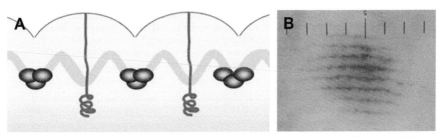

Fig. 7. Parallel furrow pattern: melanin is concentrated within the narrow furrows of plantar skin (*A*), giving rise to the parallel furrow pattern observed with the dermatoscope (*B*).

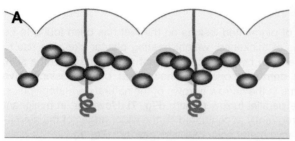
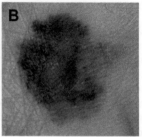

Fig. 8. (*A*) Pigment is concentrated on the wider ridges of the natural plantar dermatoglyphics (viewed at the base of the lesion). (*B*) The parallel ridge pattern as seen with the dermatoscope.

recurrence, but there is no convincing evidence that it prolongs survival. Therefore, SLNB is not universally offered in the United Kingdom. Guidelines from the United Kingdom suggest that doctors should consider using this test as a staging rather than a therapeutic procedure for people with stage 2B to 2C melanoma with a Breslow thickness of more than 1 mm.[35] As reported in one study of 84 patients with primary ALM who underwent SLNB, a positive result was more likely with thick or ulcerated ALM, and was related to a significantly shorter melanoma-specific survival (5-year survival rate, 37.5% vs 84.3%).[36]

PROGNOSIS

Tumor thickness is the most important prognostic indicator in all types of melanoma, with tumor thickness up to 1 mm being associated with a favorable prognosis.

Table 4 Melanoma staging	
Stage	**Features**
Stage 0	The melanoma is on the surface of the skin
Stage 1A	The melanoma is less than 1 mm thick
Stage 1B	The melanoma is 1–2 mm thick, or the melanoma is less than 1 mm thick and the surface of the skin is broken (ulcerated) or its cells are dividing faster than usual (mitotic activity)
Stage 2A	The melanoma is 2–4 mm thick, or the melanoma is 1–2 mm thick and is ulcerated
Stage 2B	The melanoma is thicker than 4 mm, or the melanoma is 2–4 mm thick and ulcerated
Stage 2C	The melanoma is thicker than 4 mm and ulcerated
Stage 3A	The melanoma has spread into 1–3 nearby lymph nodes, but they are not enlarged; the melanoma is not ulcerated and has not spread further
Stage 3B	The melanoma is ulcerated and has spread into 1–3 nearby lymph nodes but they are not enlarged, or the melanoma is not ulcerated and has spread into 1–3 nearby lymph nodes and they are enlarged, or the melanoma has spread to small areas of skin or lymphatic channels, but not to nearby lymph nodes
Stage 3C	The melanoma is ulcerated and has spread into 1–3 nearby lymph nodes and they are enlarged, or the melanoma has spread into 4 or more lymph nodes nearby
Stage 4	The melanoma cells have spread to other areas of the body, such as the lungs, brain, or other parts of the skin

Adapted from Levit EK, Kagen MH, Scher RK, et al. The ABC rule for clinical detection of subungual melanoma. J Am Acad Dermatol 2000;42(2 Pt 1):269–74.

However, studies have highlighted that melanomas arising on the foot have a worse prognosis than melanomas elsewhere on the body.[37] This finding may be in part caused by remote regions of the body, such as the foot, rarely being visualized and inspected by the patient and so lesions may be noticed at a more advanced stage. Moreover, even when a lesion is identified on the foot, patients may delay seeking medical attention. In one review of 27 cases of foot melanoma, the average time to seek medical attention was 13.5 months.[24]

A study of 1413 cases of ALM in the United States aligned with this suggestion, showing that only 41% of ALM cases were diagnosed with a thickness of up to 1 mm, compared with 70% of CMs at other sites. In addition, ALM had significantly poorer melanoma-specific survival rates compared with CM overall, even after controlling for thickness. This finding suggests that the lower survival rates seen in ALM may be secondary to reported different biological characteristics of the melanoma subtypes.[15]

CURRENT AND RECENT ADVANCES IN THE TREATMENT OF MELANOMA

Following confirmation of a melanoma, wide excision of the lesion, or amputation of the affected digit, and observation remain the mainstay of therapy. The width of the excision is guided by the thickness of the lesion (**Table 5**).

In patients with distant metastases, surgical management of these has been shown to be of benefit. However, recent developments in drug therapies exploiting genetic mutations have shown promise.

Genetic mutations are present in most melanomas. Different mutations are associated with specific clinical melanoma subtypes. For example, in CM, BRAF and NRAS mutations are seen in 40% to 50% and 15% to 20% of cases respectively. However, in acral and mucosal melanomas, these mutations occur in less than 10% of cases. Mutations in C-KIT are seen in approximately 15% to 20% of patients with acral or mucosal melanomas and in a smaller percentage of melanomas arising in areas of chronic skin damage.

As well as being associated with specific melanoma subtypes, the genetic mutations seen in melanoma have created new specific targeted therapies for advanced stage disease (metastatic melanoma). Tumors with BRAF mutations can be targeted with vemurafenib and dabrafenib (BRAF inhibitors), which result in progression-free survival of approximately 5 to 7 months.[38] Progression-free survival has been increased to more than 9 months when BRAF inhibitors are combined with trametinib.[39]

In order to guide treatment options for advanced melanoma, samples from metastases can be sent for genetic testing. If BRAF mutations are not detected, then treatment options include the immune checkpoint inhibitors ipilimumab and pembrolizumab.[40] The response to ipilimumab seems the same for acral melanoma

Table 5	
Excision margins for melanoma	
Tumor Thickness (mm)	**Recommended Margins (cm)**
In Situ	0.5
<2	1.0
>2	2.0

Data from Testori A, Rutkowski P, Marsden J, et al. Surgery and radiotherapy in the treatment of cutaneous melanoma. Ann Oncol 2009;20(Suppl 6):vi24.

as for other melanoma subtypes.[41] As mentioned previously, acral melanomas are more likely to express C-KIT mutation. Several phase II trials of imatinib, a KIT inhibitor, have produced mixed results and further studies are ongoing.[42]

REFERENCES

1. World Health Organization. How common is skin cancer. 2015. Available at: http://www.who.int/uv/faq/skincancer/en/index1.html. Accessed December 20, 2015.
2. Du Vries E, Bray FI, Coebergh WW, et al. Changing epidemiology of malignant cutaneous melanoma in Europe 1953-1997: rising trends in incidence and mortality but recent stabilizations in Western Europe and decreases in Scandinavia. Int J Cancer 2003;107(1):119–26.
3. Goodson AG, Grossman D. Strategies for early melanoma detection: approaches to the patient with nevi. J Am Acad Dermatol 2009;60(5):719–38.
4. Albreski D, Sloan SB. Melanoma of the feet: misdiagnosed and misunderstood. Clin Dermatol 2009;27(6):556–63.
5. Kuchelmeister C, Schaumburg-Lever G, Garbe C. Acral cutaneous melanoma in Caucasians: clinical features, histopathology and prognosis in 112 patients. Br J Dermatol 2000;143(2):275–80.
6. Feibleman CE, Stoll H, Maize JC. Melanomas of the palm, sole, and nailbed: a clinicopathologic study. Cancer 1980;46(11):2492–504.
7. Katz RD, Potter GK, Slutskiy PZ, et al. A statistical survey of melanomas of the foot. J Am Acad Dermatol 1993;28(6):1008–11.
8. Jaimes N, Braun RP, Thomas L, et al. Clinical and dermoscopic characteristics of amelanotic melanomas that are not of the nodular subtype. J Eur Acad Dermatol Venereol 2012;26(5):591–6.
9. Liu WD, Dowling JP, Murray WK, et al. Amelanotic primary cutaneous melanoma - clinical associations and dynamic evolution. Australas J Dermatol 2006;47(S1): A1–54.
10. Bristow IR, de Berker DA, Acland KM, et al. Clinical guidelines for the recognition of melanoma of the foot and nail unit. J Foot Ankle Res 2010;3:25.
11. Banfield CC, Redburn JC, Dawber RP. The incidence and prognosis of nail apparatus melanoma. A retrospective study of 105 patients in four English regions. Br J Dermatol 1998;139(2):276–9.
12. Chevalier V, Barbe C, Le Clainche A, et al. Comparison of anatomical locations of cutaneous melanoma in men and women: a population-based study in France. Br J Dermatol 2014;171(3):595–601.
13. Bellows CF, Belafsky P, Fortgang IS, et al. Melanoma in African-Americans: trends in biological behavior and clinical characteristics over two decades. J Surg Oncol 2001;78(1):10–6.
14. Jimbow K, Takahashi H, Miura S, et al. Biological behavior and natural course of acral malignant melanoma. Clinical and histologic features and prognosis of palmoplantar, subungual, and other acral malignant melanomas. Am J Dermatopathol 1984;6(Suppl):43–53.
15. Bradford PT, Goldstein AM, McMaster ML, et al. Acral lentiginous melanoma: incidence and survival patterns in the United States, 1986-2005. Arch Dermatol 2009;145(4):427–34.
16. Ragnarsson-Oldiong BK. Spatial density of primary malignant melanoma in sun-shielded body sites: a potential guide to melanoma genesis. Acta Oncol 2011;50: 323–8.

17. Parker SG, Diffey BL. The transmission of optical radiation through human nails. Br J Dermatol 1983;108(1):11–6.
18. Juzeniene A, Micu E, Porojnicu AC, et al. Malignant melanomas on head/neck and foot: differences in time and latitudinal trends in Norway. J Eur Acad Dermatol Venereol 2012;26(7):821–7.
19. Briggs JC. The role of trauma in the aetiology of malignant melanoma: a review article. Br J Plast Surg 1984;37(4):514–6.
20. Green A, McCredie M, MacKie R, et al. A case-control study of melanomas of the soles and palms (Australia and Scotland). Cancer Causes Control 1999;10(1):21–5.
21. Allen AC, Spitz S. Malignant melanoma; a clinicopathological analysis of the criteria for diagnosis and prognosis. Cancer 1953;6(1):1–45.
22. Fortes C, de Vries E. Nonsolar occupational risk factors for cutaneous melanoma. Int J Dermatol 2008;47(4):319–28.
23. Osborne JE, Bourke JF, Graham-Brown RAC, et al. False negative clinical diagnoses of malignant melanoma. Br J Dermatol 1999;140(5):902–8.
24. Bristow I, Acland K. Acral lentiginous melanoma of the foot: a review of 27 cases. J Foot Ankle Res 2008;1(1):11.
25. Fortin PT, Freiberg AA, Rees R, et al. Malignant melanoma of the foot and ankle. J Bone Joint Surg Am 1995;77(9):1396–403.
26. Dunkley MP, Morris AM. Cutaneous malignant melanoma: audit of the diagnostic process. Ann R Coll Surg Engl 1991;73(4):248–52.
27. Friedman RJ, Rigel DS, Kopf AW. Early detection of malignant melanoma: the role of physician examination and self-examination of the skin. CA Cancer J Clin 1985;35(3):130–51.
28. Argenziano G, Soyer HP. Dermoscopy of pigmented skin lesions–a valuable tool for early diagnosis of melanoma. Lancet Oncol 2001;2(7):443–9.
29. Menzies SW. Evidence-based dermoscopy. Dermatol Clin 2013;31(4):521–4, vii.
30. Argenziano G, Ferrara G, Francione S, et al. Dermoscopy–the ultimate tool for melanoma diagnosis. Semin Cutan Med Surg 2009;28(3):142–8.
31. Levit EK, Kagen MH, Scher RK, et al. The ABC rule for clinical detection of subungual melanoma. J Am Acad Dermatol 2000;42(2 Part 1):269–74.
32. Saida T, Miyazaki A, Oguchi S, et al. Significance of dermoscopic patterns in detecting malignant melanoma on acral volar skin: results of a multicenter study in Japan. Arch Dermatol 2004;140(10):1233–8.
33. Koga H, Saida T, Uhara H. Key point in dermoscopic differentiation between early nail apparatus melanoma and benign longitudinal melanonychia. J Dermatol 2011;38(1):45–52.
34. Balch CM, Gershenwald JE, Soong SJ, et al. Final version of 2009 AJCC melanoma staging and classification. J Clin Oncol 2009;27(36):6199–206.
35. National Institute for Health and Care Excellence. Melanoma: assessment and management (NG14). London: 2015. Available at: http://www.nice.org.uk/guidance/ng14. Accessed March 22, 2016.
36. Ito T, Wada M, Nagae K, et al. Acral lentiginous melanoma: who benefits from sentinel lymph node biopsy? J Am Acad Dermatol 2015;72(1):71–7.
37. Sanlorenzo M, Osella-Abate S, Ribero S, et al. Melanoma of the lower extremities: foot site is an independent risk factor for clinical outcome. Int J Dermatol 2015;54(9):1023–9.
38. McArthur GA, Chapman PB, Robert C, et al. Safety and efficacy of vemurafenib in BRAF(V600E) and BRAF(V600K) mutation-positive melanoma (BRIM-3): extended

follow-up of a phase 3, randomised, open-label study. Lancet Oncol 2014;15(3): 323–32.

39. Flaherty KT, Infante JR, Daud A, et al. Combined BRAF and MEK inhibition in melanoma with BRAF V600 mutations. N Engl J Med 2012;367(18):1694–703.

40. Robert C, Schachter J, Long GV, et al. Pembrolizumab versus ipilimumab in advanced melanoma. N Engl J Med 2015;372(26):2521–32.

41. Johnson DB, Peng C, Abramson RG, et al. Clinical activity of ipilimumab in acral melanoma: a retrospective review. Oncologist 2015;20(6):648–52.

42. Hodi FS, Corless CL, Giobbie-Hurder A, et al. Imatinib for melanomas harboring mutationally activated or amplified KIT arising on mucosal, acral, and chronically sun-damaged skin. J Clin Oncol 2013;31(26):3182–90.

Cutaneous Markers of Systemic Disease in the Lower Extremity

Joseph Vella, DPM, AACFAS

KEYWORDS

- Systemic disease • Cutaneous manifestations • Lower extremity • Skin disorders

KEY POINTS

- Many systemic diseases have cutaneous manifestations in the lower extremity, including diabetes, kidney disease, cardiovascular disorders, thyroid disease, malignancy, viral infections, genetic disorders, and even idiopathic conditions.
- These manifestations in the skin and nails of the lower extremity can not only help identify underlying conditions but can also determine treatment and prognosis.
- This article discusses a wide range of these manifestations along with their causes, helpful diagnostic tools, treatments, and prognoses.

INTRODUCTION

An old English adage gives advice that everyone is familiar with, that advice being "Don't judge a book by its cover." However, the human body is not a book, and this is evident in the way that the skin can be a window to people's health. Multiple conditions, including diabetes, kidney disease, gastrointestinal disorders, infectious processes, and even cancer can produce evidence of their arrival in the skin and nails. This article discusses the diagnosis and treatment of many of these cutaneous markers of systemic disease, particularly those that manifest in the lower extremity.

DIABETES MELLITUS
Diabetic Dermopathy

Most physicians have dealt with the effects of diabetes at some point in their careers, if not regularly. One of the most affected areas is the lower extremity, particularly with regard to neuropathy, vascular disease, and ulceration. One of the most common cutaneous manifestations of the disease is diabetic dermopathy, presenting in 40% of

Disclosure: The author has no financial disclosures and no conflict of interest to report.
Private Practice, Impression Foot & Ankle, 5656 South Power Road, Suite 124, Gilbert, AZ 85295, USA
E-mail address: JosephVellaDPM@gmail.com

patients at some point in the course of disease. It is associated with an increased likelihood of internal complications such as retinopathy, neuropathy, and nephropathy, and may be another result of microangiopathy. It begins as round, flat-topped, scaly red papules on the shins that evolve into round, atrophic hyperpigmented lesions of variable size (**Fig. 1**). Biopsy shows hemosiderin deposition, dermal edema, thickened superficial blood vessels, extravasation of erythrocytes, and a mild lymphocytic infiltrate. Although asymptomatic, these lesions can be cosmetically unpleasant, but there is no treatment available.[1,2]

Bullosis Diabeticorum

Another cutaneous manifestation of diabetes is bullosis diabeticorum, which is a rare manifestation with a reported US incidence of 0.5%. This condition consists of tense noninflamed bullae that form abruptly on the extremities, mainly the lower extremity, on the tips of the toes and soles (**Fig. 2**). They develop seemingly overnight without any history of preceding trauma and usually cause little pain or discomfort. The cause of these lesions is unknown, but microangiopathy is suspected because most patients have other diabetic complications like nephropathy and neuropathy. These bullae may be the first sign of underlying glycemic abnormalities. The disease is self-limited, usually resolving in 2 to 6 weeks without scarring as long as there is no secondary infection. Treatment simply involves compression with local wound care if necessary. Many patients never have another episode, however recurrence is not uncommon.[1,3]

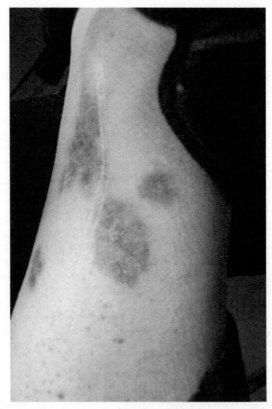

Fig. 1. Diabetic dermopathy. (*Courtesy of* Stephen Schleicher, MD, Hazleton, PA.)

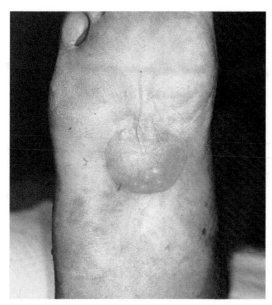

Fig. 2. Bullosis diabeticorum. (*Courtesy of* Jeff Page, DPM, Glendale, AZ.)

Diabetic Eruptive Xanthomas

Diabetic patients also develop eruptive xanthomas in the lower extremity, which present as yellow lipid deposits in the skin and tendons. Frequently they occur on extensor surfaces or on the Achilles tendon. Because they are secondary to lipid abnormalities, they can resolve on their own once the lipid levels are controlled. However, tendinous xanthomas tend to persist and may need to be surgically removed. Xanthomas are not exclusive to diabetes; they also occur with dyslipidemias, hypothyroidism, Cushing disease, alcohol usage, systemic lupus erythematosus, renal disease, liver disease, and medications such as β-blockers and estrogens.[1]

Necrobiosis Lipoidica Diabeticorum

Necrobiosis lipoidica diabeticorum is a controversial cutaneous manifestation of diabetes. It is now frequently referred to simply as necrobiosis lipoidica because it is also associated with sarcoidosis, inflammatory bowel disease, autoimmune thyroiditis, rheumatoid arthritis, and monoclonal gammopathy. Although only 0.3% to 0.7% of diabetics develop this condition, 75% of patients with necrobiosis lipoidica (NL) have or will develop diabetes mellitus eventually. The cause is unclear, although microangiopathy is the most accepted theory. It usually arises between the third and fifth decades of life on the anterior aspects of the lower legs. It begins as multiple erythematous papules that coalesce into violaceous or red-brown plaques, but it eventually morphs into a yellow-brown plaque or patches with an erythematous border, waxy/atrophic surface, and prominent telangiectasias **(Fig. 3)**.

There are no evidence-based treatment guidelines for NL because of a lack of quality randomized controlled trials. Tight glucose control has not shown benefit, thus supporting the idea that it is not as strongly associated with diabetes as was once thought. At present, steroids are the mainstay of treatment with various methods of administration, including topical, injectable, and oral. Although steroids control and possibly arrest the inflammatory process, they also promote atrophy and

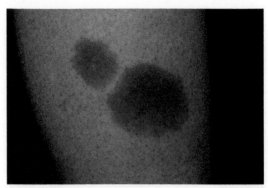

Fig. 3. Necrobiosis lipoidica diabeticorum. (*Courtesy of* Stephen Schleicher, MD, Hazleton, PA.)

hyperglycemia, so other treatment modalities have been explored, one of the most successful being pentoxifylline (Trental) at a dosage of 400 mg thrice daily for at least 6 months.[4] Other treatment modalities include immunosuppressive drugs like cyclosporine, calcineurin inhibitors, psoralen plus ultraviolet light therapy (PUVA), retinoids, hyperbaric oxygen therapy, and even skin grafting.[1,4,5]

RENAL DISEASE
Acquired Perforating Dermatosis of End-stage Renal Disease (Kyrle Disease)

Renal disease is another systemic illness that can manifest in the skin of the lower extremities, and Kyrle disease is one example. Most common in young or middle-aged African American men, Kyrle disease consists of intensely itchy dome-shaped papules on the lower extremities (**Fig. 4**). These itchy papules also have central keratotic plugs that histologically show keratin and necrotic debris. Although its main association is with kidney disease, Kyrle disease can also be seen in other conditions, such as diabetes, heart disease, and hepatitis. It may also be idiopathic, although a thorough work-up should be done to confirm this. As with most systemically derived cutaneous disorders, controlling the systemic disease can help, but resistant and idiopathic cases need topical steroids and possibly an antihistamine. There is limited evidence supporting the use of allopurinol 100 to 300 mg 3 times daily.[6] Other treatments include retinoids, vitamin A, and ultraviolet light therapy.[6–8]

Nephrogenic Fibrosing Dermopathy

Nephrogenic fibrosing dermopathy is a rare condition mostly seen in patients with severe kidney disease who were recently administered gadolinium-based contrast agents (GBCAs). The incidence of this disease has been reported as 1% to 5% in patients on chronic dialysis receiving GBCAs, as well as 10 cases in 50 million applications of GBCAs worldwide.[9,10] Its name comes from the characteristic skin lesions that patients develop, mostly on the extremities and trunk, which consist of fibrotic plaques or nodules along with a brawny texture to the skin, which has been described as peau d'orange, cobblestone, or woody. Histopathologically, these lesions show thickened collagen bundles with surrounding clefts and increased spindle-shaped cells.

However, this fibrosis does not stop at the skin, also affecting periarticular tissues, the lungs, and the heart. For this reason, the disease has been renamed nephrogenic systemic fibrosis. There is no treatment of this condition; moreover, 80% of these patients do not improve and possibly expire because of the systemic fibrosis. However, because recognition of this serious disease has become more widespread and stricter

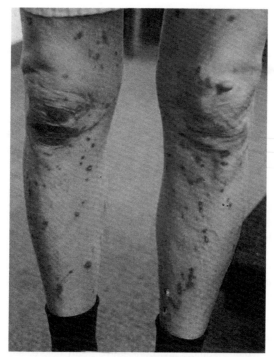

Fig. 4. Kyrle disease. (*Courtesy of* Stephen Schleicher, MD, Hazleton, PA.)

guidelines in the use of GBCAs in patients with renal disease have been implemented, nephrogenic systemic fibrosis is now rarely seen.[9–11]

Calciphylaxis

Calciphylaxis is an ischemic small vessel vasculopathy also known as calcific uremic arteriolopathy. It is seen in 1% to 4% of patients on hemodialysis, which is its main association; however, it is also seen in primary hyperparathyroidism, alcoholic liver disease, malignancy, and protein C and S deficiencies.[12] This condition manifests as extremely painful necrotic ulcers on the feet and legs (**Fig. 5**). Although usually not necessary, biopsy is the gold standard for diagnosis, and shows cutaneous necrosis, fibrin thrombi, endovascular fibrosis, and calcification. Treatment involves intravenous administration of sodium thiosulfate, usually 25 g after each dialysis session.

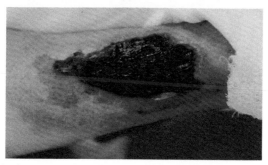

Fig. 5. Calciphylaxis. (*Courtesy of* Stephen Schleicher, MD, Hazleton, PA.)

Most patients improve temporarily, but only 25% to 30% completely resolve. Moreover, the 1-year mortality is still between 45% to 80% even with treatment.[8,12]

CARDIOVASCULAR DISORDERS
Raynaud Phenomenon

It is well known that cardiovascular disorders have effects on the extremities, and edema is not the only symptom. For example, patients with Raynaud phenomenon experience digital vasospasm, resulting in ischemia and cyanosis of the fingers and toes, which turns them red, white and blue. Although cold temperatures and stress seem to facilitate this process, the actual cause is more complicated. This condition does have an idiopathic primary version, usually in young women; however, it also has associations with a multitude of diseases, such as systemic sclerosis, systemic lupus erythematosus, dermatomyositis, Buerger disease, cryoglobulinemia, and cold agglutinin disease. Moreover, it is associated with certain drugs, such as beta-adrenergic blockers and nicotine. When it is associated with another disease, treatment of that underlying disease is the main priority. Regardless of the cause, avoiding stress, cold temperatures, and nicotine prevents recurrences. If pharmacologic treatment is necessary, calcium channel blockers and prostacyclin analogues such as iloprost have shown the most success in the literature. Other treatments include topical nitroglycerin and peripheral nerve blocks.[13–15]

Subacute Bacterial Endocarditis

Subacute bacterial endocarditis (SBE) is an infection of the endometrial surface of the heart. It causes valvular insufficiency, congestive heart failure, septicemia, embolic strokes, and even death. The classic signs of SBE include fever with a heart murmur and petechiae. Some of the lower extremity manifestations include subungual splinter hemorrhages, painful nodules on the digits (Osler nodes), and nontender maculae on the palms and soles (Janeway lesions). Diagnosis is usually made via blood cultures and echocardiogram with common signs and symptoms. Antibiotic treatment is necessary to prevent the serious complications of this condition mentioned previously.[13,16]

Henoch-Schönlein Purpura

Also known as anaphylactoid purpura, this is the most common cause of vasculitis in children, with most patients being less than the age of 10 years. It involves vascular deposition of immunoglobulin (Ig)-A–dominant immune complexes and causes such signs and symptoms as palpable purpura over the legs and buttocks (**Fig. 6**), abdominal

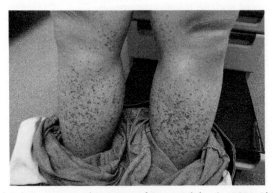

Fig. 6. Henoch-Schönlein purpura. (*Courtesy of* Tracey Vlahovic, DPM, Philadelphia, PA.)

pain, gastrointestinal bleeding, arthralgia, nephritis, and hematuria. On histology it shows a leukocytoclastic vasculitis. The cause is unknown; however, it is strongly believed that genetic predisposition mixed with environmental factors (such as infection, which is a precipitating factor in at least 50% of patients) promotes development of this condition.[17] Usually Henoch-Schönlein purpura is self-limited, only requiring symptomatic treatment; however, one-third of patients have 1 or more recurrences. Moreover, the prognosis of this condition is linked to kidney function, which can be severely affected; therefore, monitoring kidney function is essential, and immunomodulators such as steroids or cyclosporine may be necessary to mitigate the damage to the kidneys.[1,17,18]

THYROID CONDITIONS
Thyroid Dermopathy (Pretibial Myxedema)

This lower extremity cutaneous manifestation is associated with Graves disease, and it consists of fleshy, yellowish-brown waxy nodules with lymphedema and the concurrent peau d'orange appearance of the skin, mainly in the pretibial region. Some investigators have described it as being elephantiasis-like edema or as having a pigskin appearance (**Fig. 7**).[8] Most patients also have thyroid ophthalmopathy, which together with the hyperthyroidism often overshadows the lower extremity changes. Dependency plays a significant role in the development of these lesions, which is why the lower extremity is mainly where it manifests. Smoking also is a significant contributing factor. The diagnosis is mostly clinical but a biopsy can resolve any doubt; it shows an accumulation of glycosaminoglycans in the reticular dermis. Usually these lesions are asymptomatic and only of cosmetic concern, although rarely they can be painful and pruritic. Treatment consists of compression and topical steroids under occlusion. Smoking cessation and weight loss to reduce dependency can help.[19]

MALIGNANCY

Certain cancers can present with cutaneous markers, even in the lower extremity. These conditions are called cutaneous paraneoplastic syndromes, and because

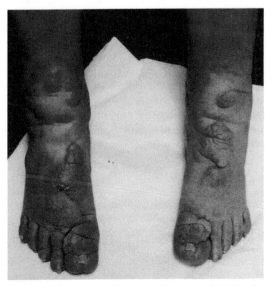

Fig. 7. Pretibial myxedema. (*Courtesy of* Stephen Schleicher, MD, Hazleton, PA.)

they correspond with internal malignancy, they can be used to measure remission or recurrence of disease. They are the result of the production of biologically active hormones or growth factors, or antigen-antibody interactions induced or produced by the tumor. There are many cutaneous paraneoplastic syndromes; only those most frequently seen in the lower extremity are discussed here.

Bazex Syndrome

Also known as acrodermatitis/acrokeratosis paraneoplastica, this cutaneous paraneoplastic syndrome is associated mostly with squamous cell carcinoma of the upper aerodigestive tract. Cutaneous manifestations consist of psoriasiform lesions of the hands, feet, nose, and ear that eventually spread to the proximal extremities and trunk. In addition, patients may develop nail dystrophy and cyanotic discoloration of the digits. As with other paraneoplastic syndromes, resection of the cancer facilitates resolution of the skin lesions, and their recurrence suggests return of the cancer.[1,13,20]

Glucagonoma Syndrome

Glucagonoma syndrome is a migratory necrolytic erythema in the intertriginous folds of the dependent areas of the body (ie, the groin, abdomen, buttocks, and lower extremities). As its name implies, it is associated with a glucagon-secreting alpha-cell tumor of the pancreas. Patients present with dry or fissured erythema, superficial flaccid vesicles, and bullae that create extensive erosions and crusted plaques after rupturing. Resection of the tumor causes rapid resolution of the erythema.[20]

Malignant Acanthosis Nigricans

Unlike its benign relative which is associated with obesity and insulin resistance, malignant acanthosis nigricans occurs when a tumor secretes products with activity similar to insulin or transforming growth factor alpha, which stimulates keratinocytes to proliferate. The most common site of the tumor is the stomach. Although benign acanthosis nigricans mostly affects the axillary and neck regions, its malignant counterpart causes velvety hyperpigmentation/hyperkeratosis on the mucous membranes, palms, and soles. In addition, the lesions are more extensive and develop more rapidly. It is also common for the lesions to cause severe itching.[1]

Ichthyosis

Ichthyosis is a congenital disorder with multiple variations, known well for the collodion baby with which it is sometimes associated. It involves scaling of the skin, giving it a fish-scale appearance, mostly prominent on the trunk and extremities. Although the inherited form is more common in children, the acquired form presents mostly in adults because of its link to cancers of the lung, breast, cervix, and lymphatics.[1]

Palmoplantar Keratoderma

The palmoplantar keratodermas, like ichthyosis, are a heterogenous group of disorders that have both congenital and cancerous origins. As the name suggests, this is a disorder of hyperkeratosis on the palmar and plantar surfaces. Although treatment of the condition mainly consists of debridement and topical keratolytics/emollients, its sudden emergence in an older patient requires work-up to rule out any underlying malignancy, such as breast, lung, gastric, leukemia, lymphoma, and thyroid.[1]

Trousseau Syndrome

Trousseau syndrome is an acquired hypercoagulability with recurrent superficial thrombophlebitis in the arterial or venous system, specifically in the trunk or extremities. Thus the patients present with recurrent tender erythematous cords or nodules caused by the clotting of the superficial vessels. This syndrome is associated with cancer 50% of the time, mostly lung and pancreatic. Therefore, prompt work-up in any patient is warranted to make an early diagnosis which, it is hoped, will facilitate a better outcome.[1]

Werner Syndrome

Although there is a rare autosomal recessive version of this condition, the acquired version is associated with fibrosarcoma of the mediastinum and multiple basal cell carcinoma. It causes premature aging with all of its less desirable effects: cataracts, short stature, greying hair/baldness, laryngeal atrophy, distal muscle atrophy, and endocrine disorders such as diabetes and osteoporosis. The skin is also affected, because it becomes dry, atrophic, and callused, particularly over bony prominences. It resembles scleroderma, and patients even develop chronic leg ulcers because of the diminished quality of the skin.[20]

GENETIC DISORDERS
Neurofibromatosis

Neurofibromatosis is a family of disorders with the most common variation being a mutation of the NF1 gene on chromosome 17. Fifty percent of the time this is a spontaneous mutation in individuals with no family history of the disease. It is the most common mutation in humans, with a worldwide incidence of 1 in 3000.[21] It is derived from neural crest cells and causes tumors surrounding the nerves in the skin, central nervous system, bone, and endocrine glands. In the skin, this results in café au lait spots, axillary freckling, Lisch nodules (iris hamartomas), and neurofibromas. The neurofibromas in particular can be troublesome and require excision, especially in the rare case (2%) of malignant transformation. Internal complications are no less significant, with patients commonly developing optic gliomas, scoliosis, and even learning disabilities. There are even reports of pseudoarthroses in certain bones, such as the tibia and radius. Regarding treatment, the cutaneous neurofibromas can be excised, but they are frequently too numerous to afford complete resolution. Genetic counseling becomes important in these cases, especially to affected couples wishing to start a family.[1]

Tuberous Sclerosis

An autosomal dominant disease, tuberous sclerosis consists of multiple hamartomas of the skin, central nervous system, kidneys, heart, retina, and gastrointestinal tract. Mental retardation is present in less than 50% of patients. Skin lesions include yellow-pink papules on the face (adenoma sebaceum), flesh-colored to yellow-colored patches in the lumbosacral region (shagreen patch), hypomelanotic patches on the trunk and extremities (ash leaf macule), and periungual fibromas (**Fig. 8**). Even though this is an autosomal dominant disease, two-thirds of cases arise sporadically. It is caused by a mutation in the TSC1 or TSC2 gene. As in neurofibromatosis, genetic counseling is important because there is a 50% chance of passing this condition on to offspring. For the skin lesions, excision is the treatment of choice.[1,8]

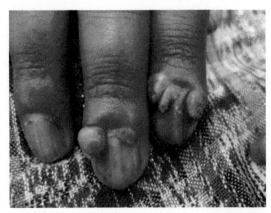

Fig. 8. Periungual fibromas in tuberous sclerosis. (*Courtesy of* Jeff Page, DPM, Glendale, AZ.)

THE ERYTHEMAS

There are multiple erythematous disorders of the lower extremities, and they usually have multiple associations, causing them to range from inconsequential to urgent. Frequently they are idiopathic, which in this case is usually comforting. However, they require work-up to rule out more serious underlying disease.

Erythema Multiforme

This is a common acute inflammatory disease that is idiopathic 50% of the time; however, it is also associated with systemic illness such as upper respiratory tract and herpes simplex infections. Patients present with targets lesions and papules on the backs of the hands and feet, as well as the extensor aspect of the forearms and legs (**Fig. 9**). These lesions may or may not cause discomfort. When biopsied, histopathology shows a mononuclear cell infiltrate in the upper dermal blood vessels. The disease is usually self-limited, and therefore mild cases need no treatment. More severe cases benefit from a 1-week to 3-week course of prednisone. Other treatments include dapsone and azathioprine.[1]

Erythema Nodosum

Erythema nodosum is a painful nodular erythematous eruption usually limited to the extensor aspects of the extremities (**Fig. 10**). As with erythema multiforme, it is idiopathic most of the time (55%). However, the list of conditions with which it is associated is more extensive, including certain infections (upper respiratory tract,

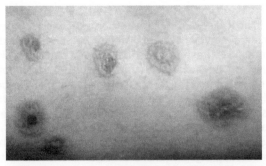

Fig. 9. Erythema multiforme. (*Courtesy of* Stephen Schleicher, MD, Hazleton, PA.)

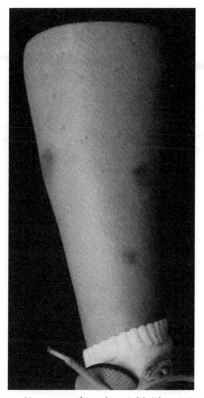

Fig. 10. Erythema nodosum. (*Courtesy of* Stephen Schleicher, MD, Hazleton, PA.)

streptococcus, coccidioidomycosis), systemic illnesses (inflammatory bowel disease, sarcoidosis), medications (sulfonamides), pregnancy, and malignancies (Hodgkin). Along with the characteristic skin lesions, patients also experience fatigue, malaise, low-grade fever, and arthralgias. As with erythema multiforme, this condition is self-limited in most cases and requires only supportive treatment. Resistant cases may require steroids, although this may worsen infections.[1]

Erythema Annulare Centrifugum

Also known as erythema perstans, erythema annulare centrifugum (EAC) is a mostly benign inflammatory dermatitis affecting both male and female patients at any age. Patients typically present with erythematous arcuate or annular patches on the lower extremities, which may or may not be pruritic and scaly (**Fig. 11**). Biopsy shows perivascular infiltrate of lymphohistiocytes, sometimes with a so-called coat-sleeve pattern. The cause is still unclear, but reported associations include certain medications (gold, antimalarial compounds), infections (eg, tuberculosis), malignancies, and stress. Some investigators have theorized that it is a delayed-type hypersensitivity caused by interaction of inflammatory mediators. In any event, EAC is normally self-limited, and therefore only requires symptomatic treatment. Steroids have been used; however, exacerbation after discontinuation of the steroid and recurrence were common. Other immunomodulators have been used with varying success, including etanercept and metronidazole. One study, by Chuang and colleagues,[22] found success with erythromycin; however, the study was small and the results vague.

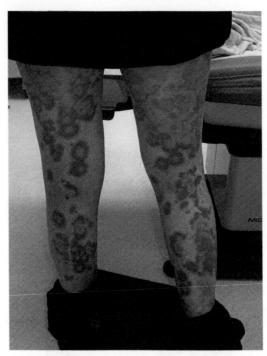

Fig. 11. Erythema annulare centrifugum. (*Courtesy of* Stephen Schleicher, MD, Hazleton, PA.)

Thorough work-up is required to rule out underlying conditions, whose treatment and resolution should facilitate clearing of EAC.[8]

Palmoplantar Erythema

Also known as chemotherapy-induced acral erythema or hand-foot syndrome, this erythematous disorder consists of well-demarcated erythema of the hands and feet after administration of certain chemotherapeutic medications (**Fig. 12**). Average onset is 2 to 21 days, although it may occur up to 10 months later with certain agents.[23] The most common associated medications include capecitabine, cytarabine, fluorouracil, docetaxel, and doxorubicin. Patients may also experience dysesthesias, edema, fissuring, and ulceration, along with stomatitis. A dose reduction or temporary discontinuation of the chemotherapy drug promotes resolution of the rash; additionally, concomitant administration of dexamethasone mitigates the reaction.[8] Other possible therapies include topical steroids, urea cream, and even cooling of the extremities.[23]

MISCELLANEOUS DISORDERS
Keratoderma Blennorrhagicum

Keratoderma blennorrhagicum is commonly associated with reactive arthritis and consists of psoriasiform patches with a scaly scalloped-edge border on the soles of the feet and toes, legs, hands, and scalp. In addition, the nails are dystrophic, although there is no pitting as in psoriasis. As mentioned earlier, this condition is associated with reactive arthritis, so patients are likely to have concurrent arthritis, urethritis, and conjunctivitis. The underlying infection must be treated, and usually this facilitates resolution of the cutaneous manifestation. However, persistent patches may require treatment with a retinoid or ketoconazole.[1]

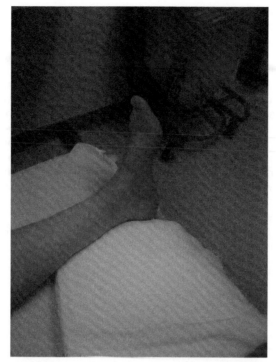

Fig. 12. Palmoplantar erythema. (*Courtesy of* Stephen Schleicher, MD, Hazleton, PA.)

Pyoderma Gangrenosum

Pyoderma gangrenosum (PG) is a rare, poorly understood ulcerating skin disease with multiple associations, the best known being inflammatory bowel disease. Of the 50% to 60% of nonidiopathic cases, ulcerative colitis is the associated illness 50% of the time. Other associated conditions include rheumatoid arthritis, chronic active hepatitis, Crohn disease, IgA monoclonal gammopathy, and hematological malignancies. PG begins as a tender erythematous nodule that progresses to a necrotic/fibrotic ulceration with violaceous rolled edges and a halo of surrounding erythema (**Fig. 13**). In 20% to 30% of patients, trauma or pathergy may precede

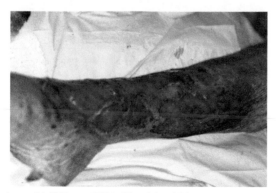

Fig. 13. PG. (*Courtesy of* Jeff Page, DPM, Glendale, AZ.)

the ulceration, and further trauma only encourages the process. The lower leg is the most common site; however, there have been reports of this condition in other locations, such as stoma sites.

There are no good diagnostic tests for PG; even histopathology is nonspecific, showing everything from folliculitis and abscess formation to vasculitis and suppurative granulomatous dermatitis. Thus it is mostly a clinical diagnosis, and a difficult one considering that the treatment of this disease goes against usual wound principles. For example, a standard wound requires debridement to bring the wound out of the chronic inflammatory stage into a more acute stage; however, inflammation and pathergy are the problem in PG, and therefore antiinflammatory measures are taken. Systemic steroids are the treatment of choice, although there is literature supporting topical and intralesional steroids as well.[24] Other immunomodulators have also been used with success, particularly cyclosporine and infliximab (Remicade, Janssen Biotech). Steroid-sparing agents such as tacrolimus and pimecrolimus in ointment form are useful for localized lesions; it has been suggested that topical tacrolimus be the first-line therapy for localized idiopathic lesions with confirmed negative microbiological tests.[24] In particularly severe cases, excision and/or grafting may be necessary; however, appropriate local wound care is always recommended.[1,8]

Vitiligo

Vitiligo is a disorder of pigmentation of unknown cause but with multiple associations, including endocrine disorders (thyroid disorders, diabetes mellitus, Addison disease), autoimmune syndromes, pernicious anemia, and even melanoma. Although it is only present in 1% of the population, 50% occurs before the age of 20 years, affecting male and female patients equally. Patients experience both localized and generalized loss of pigment, particularly in the intertriginous areas and orifices of the body (**Fig. 14**). The hands and feet are affected, along with the face and mucous membranes. Although vitiligo is benign, it has emotional and social effects that frequently motivate patients to seek treatment. Physicians should rule out underlying disorders, particularly with the thyroid because as many as 30% of patients with thyroid disorders develop vitiligo. Treatment of this condition is difficult; even the best treatment (narrow-band ultraviolet B and PUVA) requires 6 to 12 months for complete cure, even with concomitant topical steroid use.[1] A recent article in the *Journal of the American Academy of Dermatology* described a new method of treatment consisting of intralesional injections of low-dose

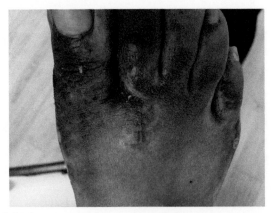

Fig. 14. Vitiligo of the foot.

steroid (3–5 mg of Kenalog), with which they had great success; however, it was a small study and further, larger randomized controlled trials are necessary to prove efficacy.[25]

NAIL MANIFESTATIONS OF INTERNAL DISEASE

No compilation of cutaneous manifestations of systemic disease would be complete without discussing nail disorders. The nails can provide many clues to physicians when making a diagnosis and planning treatment thereof. Although the manifestations discussed here are not comprehensive, they may help podiatric physicians to determine why antifungals are not working.

Beau Lines

These are transverse depressions of all the nails at the base of lunula resulting from a stressful event that temporarily interrupted nail formation. They are associated with such conditions as syphilis, uncontrolled diabetes mellitus, myocarditis, peripheral vascular disease, zinc deficiency, illnesses accompanied by high fevers (scarlet fever, measles, mumps, hand-foot-and-mouth disease, pneumonia), and chemotherapeutic agents. Although cosmetically displeasing, these lines have little significance and grow out uneventfully with the nail.[1]

Yellow Nail Syndrome

Yellow nail syndrome is a disorder of yellow nails. It has multiple associations, including lymphedema, infections (pneumonia, acquired immunodeficiency syndrome), autoimmune disorders (thyroiditis, rheumatoid arthritis), malignancy (mycosis fungoides, laryngeal carcinoma, gallbladder carcinoma, bronchial carcinoma, breast cancer, non-Hodgkin lymphoma, endometrial cancer), and other lung disorders such as pleural effusions and bronchiectasis.[10] Nail growth is slowed in this disorder as well. Treating the underlying disorder usually facilitates resolution of the nail abnormality, particularly in the case of malignancy. The yellow nails spontaneously improve in half of patients even if the underlying disease does not. For resistant cases, vitamin E may be required, either 800 IU/d orally or drops of a 5% solution twice a day.[1]

Koilonychia

Koilonychia, or spoon nails (**Fig. 15**), is a normal occurrence in children. It may persist for a lifetime without any associated abnormality. New cases in adults may be associated with iron deficiency anemia and idiopathic hemochromatosis; therefore, a work-up is warranted. Like most secondary conditions, it clears up with resolution of the primary disease.[1]

Digital Clubbing

Also known as Hippocratic nails, this disorder can be either a normal variant or associated with serious underlying disease. It is only painful in hypertrophic osteoarthropathy. All patients with cyanotic congenital heart disease develop clubbing as well as one-third of lung patients with cancer. In North America, 80% of acquired digital clubbing is associated with pulmonary disease. Other associations include cirrhosis, colitis, and thyroid disease. This deformity is usually permanent, even with resolution or control of the underlying disease (**Fig. 16**).[1]

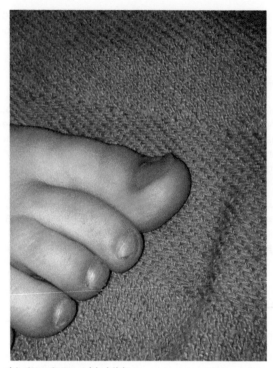

Fig. 15. K koilonychia in a 6-year-old child.

Terry Nails

Patients with Terry nails present with proximal nail whitening that makes it difficult to distinguish the lunula (**Fig. 17**). This whitening is caused by decreased capillary blood flow to the nail bed, which is caused by increased growth of underlying connective tissue. It is mostly seen in patients with severe liver disease, but other associated conditions include congestive heart failure, diabetes, increasing age, and malnutrition. Treatment is designed to address the underlying condition.[13]

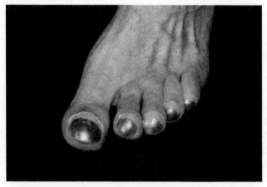

Fig. 16. Digital clubbing. (*Courtesy of* Tracey Vlahovic, DPM, Philadelphia, PA.)

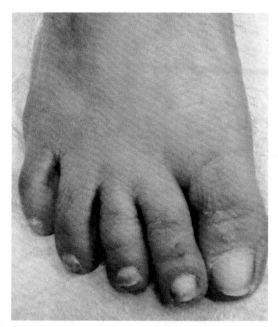

Fig. 17. Terry nails. (*Courtesy of* Tracey Vlahovic, DPM, Philadelphia, PA.)

SUMMARY

The skin can be one of the most important tools in the diagnosis of systemic disease, and podiatric physicians can use this to achieve better overall outcomes in their patients. Although this list of conditions is not exhaustive, it represents a large portion of the most common cutaneous manifestations of systemic disease seen in the lower extremity. In addition, the treatment methods reviewed earlier represent the most accepted and researched algorithms, along with a discussion of future treatments. It is hoped that further research will continue to provide insights into these diseases, more effective ways of treating them, and improved quality of life for patients.

REFERENCES

1. Habif TP. Cutaneous manifestations of internal disease. In: Clinical dermatology: a color guide to diagnosis and therapy. 5th edition. (China): Mosby, Elsevier; 2010. p. 974–98.
2. Finucane KA, Archer CB. Recent advances in diabetology: diabetic dermopathy, autoantibodies in the prediction of the development of type 1 diabetes, and islet cell transplantation and inhaled insulin as treatment for diabetes. Clin Exp Dermatol 2006;31(6):837–40.
3. Bhutani R, Walton S. Diabetic bullae. Br J Diabetes Vasc Dis 2015;15:8–10.
4. Feily A, Mehraban S. Treatment modalities of necrobiosis lipoidica: a concise systematic review. Dermatol Reports 2015;7(2):5749.
5. Reid SD, Ladizinski B, Lee K, et al. Update on necrobiosis lipoidica: a review of etiology, diagnosis, and treatment options. J Am Acad Dermatol 2013;69(5):783–91.
6. Shih C, Tsai T, Huang H, et al. Kyrle's disease successfully treated with allopurinol. Int J Dermatol 2011;50:1170–2.

7. Saray Y, Seckin D, Bilezikci B. Acquired perforating dermatosis: clinicopatholog-ical features in twenty-two cases. J Eur Acad Dermatol Venereol 2006;20:679–88.
8. Vlahovic T, Schleicher SM. Skin disease of the lower extremities: a photographic guide. Malvern (PA): HMP Communications; 2012.
9. Haemel AK, Sadowski EA, Shafer MM, et al. Update on nephrogenic systemic fibrosis: are we making progress? Int J Dermatol 2011;50:659–66.
10. Heverhagen JT, Krombach GA, Gizewski E. Application of extracellular gadolinium-based MRI contrast agents and the risk of nephrogenic systemic fibrosis. Rofo 2014;186:661–9.
11. Freed L, Hill J, Gooch D. Nephrogenic systemic fibrosis in the podiatric patient. J Am Podiatr Med Assoc 2012;102(5):419–21.
12. Nigwekar SU, Brunelli SM, Meade D, et al. Sodium thiosulfate therapy for calcific uremic arteriolopathy. Clin J Am Soc Nephrol 2013;8(7):1162–70.
13. Patel LM, Lambert PF, Gagna CE, et al. Cutaneous signs of systemic disease. Clin Dermatol 2011;29(5):511–22.
14. Huisstede BM, Hoogvliet P, Paulis WD, et al. Effectiveness of interventions for secondary Raynaud's phenomenon: a systematic review. Arch Phys Med Rehabil 2011;92:1166–80.
15. Henness S, Wigley FM. Current drug therapy for scleroderma and secondary Raynaud's phenomenon: evidence-based review. Curr Opin Rheumatol 2007; 19:611–8.
16. Brusch JL. Infective endocarditis. Available at: Medscape.com. Accessed September 7, 2015.
17. He X, Yu C, Zhao P, et al. The genetics of Henoch-SchÖnlein purpura: a system-atic review and meta-analysis. Rheumatol Int 2013;33:1387–95.
18. Weiss PF, Feinstein JA, Luan X, et al. Effects of corticosteroids on Henoch-SchÖnlein purpura: a systematic review. Pediatrics 2007;120(5):1079–87.
19. Fatourechi V. Pretibial myxedema: pathophysiology and treatment options. Am J Clin Dermatol 2005;6(5):295–309.
20. Velez AMA, Howard MS. Diagnosis and treatment of cutaneous paraneoplastic disorders. Dermatol Ther 2010;23(6):662–75.
21. Hirbe AC, Gutmann DH. Neurofibromatosis type 1: a multi-disciplinary approach to care. Lancet Neurol 2014;13:834–43.
22. Chuang F, Lin S, Wu W. Erythromycin as a safe and effective treatment option for erythema annulare centrifugum. Indian J Dermatol 2015;60(5):519.
23. Miller KK, Gorcey L, McLellan BL. Chemotherapy-induced hand-foot syndrome and nail changes: a review of clinical presentation, etiology, pathogenesis, and management. J Am Acad Dermatol 2014;71:787–94.
24. Wollina U, Haroske G. Pyoderma gangraenosum. Curr Opin Rheumatol 2011;23: 50–6.
25. Wang E, Koo J, Levy E. Intralesional corticosteroid injections for vitiligo: a new therapeutic option. J Am Acad Dermatol 2014;71(2):391–3.

Plantar Hyperhidrosis

An Overview

Tracey C. Vlahovic, DPM, FFPM RCPS (Glasg)

KEYWORDS

- Plantar hyperhidrosis • Botulinum toxin • Pitted keratolysis • Tinea pedis

KEY POINTS

- Plantar hyperhidrosis affects the quality of life for patients.
- The source of hyperhidrosis should be investigated before initiating treatment.
- Various pharmacologic and nonpharmacologic treatments exist, but many offer temporary solutions.

INTRODUCTION

Plantar hyperhidrosis is excessive sweat production on the soles of the feet.[1] This condition is not caused by an increased number of sweat glands, but rather by hyperactivity of the eccrine sweat glands despite a normal body temperature.[1] It is excessive sweating disproportionate to the environmental conditions or what is needed for thermoregulation.[2]

In general, hyperhidrosis affects about 3% of the population, which does not including unreported cases, many of which may be because of patients' embarrassment.[1] Hyperhidrosis occurs at locations with a high density of eccrine glands, such as plantar, palmar, and craniofacial surfaces, and also with apocrine glands, such as in the axilla.[3] Hyperhidrosis is a condition that can affect a significant amount of years of a person's life. In the study by Walling,[3] 24.8% reported that they had it their whole life. Other than females having a slightly higher likelihood of having axillary hyperhidrosis, there have not been found to be significant gender differences in prevalence in any other anatomic site.[3,4] In a study by Lear and colleagues,[5] although there was not a difference in presentation of plantar hyperhidrosis between men and women in the American clinic, there were significantly more females presenting with plantar hyperhidrosis than males in the Canadian clinic; however, it was still a similar percentage to that of American women. The age of onset for plantar hyperhidrosis tends to be between 0 and 19 years, with almost 56% occurring between 0 and 11 years.[5] It has

Disclosure: The author has nothing to disclose.
Department of Podiatric Medicine, Temple University School of Podiatric Medicine, 148 North 8th Street, Philadelphia, PA 19107, USA
E-mail address: traceyv@temple.edu

Clin Podiatr Med Surg 33 (2016) 441–451
http://dx.doi.org/10.1016/j.cpm.2016.02.010
0891-8422/16/$ – see front matter © 2016 Elsevier Inc. All rights reserved.

been suggested that hyperhidrosis may regress spontaneously over time because of the low prevalence among the elderly.[5] Almost 47% had primary hyperhidrosis of multiple sites, and plantar hyperhidrosis was present in just over 50% of cases, making it the most frequently involved anatomic site.[3] In an epidemiologic study by Lear and colleagues,[5] the plantar surface of the foot was affected in almost 46% of patients with hyperhidrosis. In a study of 447 medical students in the State of Sergipe, Brazil, 25% had plantar hyperhidrosis.[5] Hyperhidrosis is a generalized condition with various etiologies, but when it is focal, such as it is when it solely affects the plantar surface of feet, it is usually idiopathic.[1] However, some other causes of focal hyperhidrosis include malignancy, or congenital/genetic causes, such as epidermolysis bullosa syndromes, pachyonychia congenital, palmoplantar keratoderma syndromes, or eccrine gland autonomic pathologies.[2]

PATIENT EVALUATION OVERVIEW

Plantar hyperhidrosis is typically primary hyperhidrosis and idiopathic, but hyperhidrosis is divided into primary and secondary categories.[2] Primary hyperhidrosis tends to be an idiopathic increase in sympathetic nervous system activity; secondary usually is caused by either a medication or an underlying disease.[2] In the study by Walling[2] of 415 patients, 93.3% had primary and the remaining 6.7% had secondary. Primary hyperhidrosis tends to be typically distributed in the axilla, palms, soles, and craniofacial area in a bilateral and symmetric pattern, with an increase in cutaneous infections.[2] In this study, 25% of those with primary hyperhidrosis had palms and soles affected; 15.5% had just soles; and 11% had axilla, palms, and soles. Thus, 51.5% of those with primary were affected by hyperhidrosis on the soles of their feet. Although secondary hyperhidrosis does affect the feet, it has different etiologies and typical patterns of distribution.[2] Secondary hyperhidrosis tends to be caused by generalized medical conditions or medications.[2] The generalized medical conditions include endocrine, neurologic, cardiovascular, neoplastic, and infectious diseases.[2] A total of 57% of those with secondary hyperhidrosis were caused by endocrine pathology, including diabetes mellitus, hyperthyroidism, and hyperpituitarism, and 32% were caused by neurologic diseases including peripheral nerve injury, Parkinson disease, reflex sympathetic dystrophy, spinal cord injury, and Arnold-Chiari malformation.[2] When evaluating a patient with excessive plantar sweating, the clinician should ascertain if laboratory testing for the thyroid has been done. If it has not, it is imperative to do so before proceeding to the more invasive and systemic therapies. Secondary is more likely to be unilateral and/or asymmetrically distributed, generalized more than focal, to be present at night during sleep, to have an onset older than age 25, and is more likely to lack a family history of the condition.[2] The medications that may cause secondary hyperhidrosis are adrenergics, anticholinesterases/cholinergics, antidepressants, antidiabetic agents, antiemetics, antineoplastics, antipsychotics, antipyretics, anxiolytics, alcohol, and opiates.[2]

Because patients range from having visible sweating to a palpable moistness, the diagnosis of primary focal hyperhidrosis is not simply excessive sweating.[6] The criteria for diagnosis generally is excessive sweating that lasts for at least 6 months and has at least two of the following symptoms: a bilateral and symmetric pattern of sweating that occurs at least once per week, impairs daily activities, started before the age of 25, focal sweating stops during sleep at night, a score of 3 or 4 on the Hyperhidrosis Disease Severity Scale (HDSS; **Box 1**), and a family history.[7] The HDSS may be given to the patient in written or verbal form and represents a simple and easy to understand way of relating the disease state to daily activities. It is a scale of 1 to 4,

---

Box 1
Hyperhidrosis disease severity scale

When rating the severity of plantar hyperhidrosis the patient is experiencing, ask the patient which number characterizes the situation.

1. My foot sweating is never noticeable and never interferes with my daily activities.

2. My foot sweating is tolerable but sometimes interferes with my daily activities.

3. My foot sweating is barely tolerable and frequently interferes with my daily activities.

4. My foot sweating is intolerable and always interferes with my daily activities.

Adapted from Solish N, Bertucci V, Dansereau A, et al. A comprehensive approach to the recognition, diagnosis, and severity-based treatment of focal hyperhidrosis: recommendations of the Canadian Hyperhidrosis Advisory Committee. Dermatol Surg 2007;33(8):910; with permission.

---

with 4 describing the sweating as "intolerable and always interfering with daily activities." Because many podiatric patients may complain of changing socks frequently, malodor, and difficulty finding shoes that do not make them sweat, the practitioner may add asking those questions and the HDSS (**Box 2**). If the patient is experiencing a full body presentation, Walling[2] described a more specific diagnostic criterion with a higher positive predicative value in determining the presence of primary hyperhidrosis. He defined it as excessive sweating for 6 months or more with four of the following: presence in eccrine-dense areas, such as axilla, palms, soles, and craniofacial; bilateral and symmetric distribution; absent nocturnally; episodes at least weekly; onset of 25 years or younger; family history; and the impairment of daily activities.[2]

Box 2
Evaluation of a patient with plantar hyperhidrosis

A thorough history and physical should be completed that includes evaluating the following:

Has there been plantar excessive sweating greater than 6 months?

Is it bilateral and relatively symmetric? Or is it unilateral?

The HDSS score (see **Box 1**); greater than 3 or 4 is diagnostic.

Age of onset less than 25 years/family history.

Cessation of plantar sweating during sleep?

Do you have excessive sweating anywhere else besides your feet?

Have you been tested for thyroid disease, diabetes, or are on any medications that have changed your sweating frequency since you started taking them?

How many times a day do you change your socks?

Do you worry about wearing sandals because you will walk out of your shoes from sweat?

Does sweat ruin your shoes?

Does sweating interfere with playing sports?

Is your feet cold in the winter or in air conditioning because of sweating?

Is there any odor and does anything help to make it better?

Have you or has anyone diagnosed you with athlete's foot (tinea pedis)?

Are there warts, pitted keratolysis, or erythrasma present (a Wood lamp assists with diagnosing erythrasma).

There is some evidence that primary hyperhidrosis is an autosomal-dominant trait with variable penetrance.[8,9] In a study of 410 patients in Japan, 36% had positive family histories of palmoplantar hyperhidrosis.[9] The most common pattern was parent-child (58%) incidence, and 13% of patients had three generations affected by palmoplantar hyperhidrosis.[9] In Lear and colleagues,[5] almost 44% reported a relative with hyperhidrosis. In the study by Lima and coworders[4] of 447 medical students, 45% reported a family history of the condition.

There are various conditions that can complicate plantar hyperhidrosis. It is an embarrassing condition that unfortunately people tend to delay seeking care for, even delaying it up to almost 9 years from the onset of symptoms.[3] Mood changes, such as anxiety and embarrassment, are associated with hyperhidrosis.[10] Activities, such as sports, and professional and interpersonal relationships can all be affected because shoes and socks may need to be changed several times per day.[4,10,11] Braganca and colleagues[10] investigated the prevalence of anxiety and depression in people with primary hyperhidrosis, and found that the prevalence of anxiety, more so than depression, is significantly increased compared with the general population. Seventy-two percent had the plantar surfaces affected, and 68% of those with anxiety had plantar hyperhidrosis. Of those with just the plantar surfaces affected, 13% had bromhidrosis and a third of them had anxiety. Many people with plantar hyperhidrosis develop bromhidrosis, which is an unpleasant odor caused by the decomposition of sweat by bacteria.[12] In a study by Ak and colleagues,[6] people with primary focal hyperhidrosis reported lower levels of purposefulness, resourcefulness, and self-directedness, and higher levels of self-forgetfulness. Not only can hyperhidrosis cause emotional stress, in Walling's[3] case control study in 2009, he found that 56.7% of the patients with primary hyperhidrosis reported that it was exacerbated by stress, emotion, anxiety, or social situations. In Lima and coworkers,[4] 78% also reported that the condition was exacerbated by stress. In addition, 22% percent of people reported that it was also exacerbated by heat and humidity.[3]

The overall risk of any cutaneous infection was increased in sites with hyperhidrosis.[3] There is an increased risk of fungal infections, with a particularly increased risk of dermatophyte infections of cutaneous surfaces, such as tinea pedis, tinea manuum, tinea corporis, and tinea cruris.[3] In patients with onychomycosis and hyperhidrosis, maceration of the skin decreases the defense against fungal infection, and the damp environment facilitates the growth and proliferation of fungi.[13] In a study by Zheng and colleagues,[13] out of 40 cases of patients with both onychomycosis and hyperhidrosis, 20 were treated for onychomycosis, and the other 20 were treated for both onychomycosis and hyperhidrosis. Sixteen out of 20 just treated for onychomycosis were cured, but 20 out of 20 treated for both onychomycosis and hyperhidrosis were cured. In a German case control study of 30 patients with tinea pedis, they had a 3.5-fold higher rate of hyperhidrosis than those without tinea pedis.[14] With hyperhidrosis, there is also an increased risk of bacterial infection, particularly pitted keratolysis.[3] The presence of hyperhidrosis and other symptoms, such as maceration, is seen in 70% to 90% of cases of pitted keratolysis.[15] Although pitted keratolysis is treated successfully with topical medications, it can also be very resistant to treatment and chronically recur in the presence of hyperhidrosis or bromidrosis.[15] The presence of hyperhidrosis in pitted keratolysis may either create a supportive environment for bacterial growth and proliferation, or it may lessen the effect of topical medications.[15] An Italian study by Pranteda and colleagues[16] in 2014 sought to investigate varying hypotheses regarding the relationship between pitted keratolysis and hyperhidrosis. One hypothesis suggests that the presence of hyperhidrosis is a predisposing factor for bacterial infection and growth, whereas another suggests that hyperhidrosis may in fact be the result, rather than the cause, of bacterial infection.[16] In this study, erythromycin 3% topical gel was applied twice daily without concurrent treatment of hyperhidrosis, and gravimetric measurements were taken of plantar sweating. Before treatment 94 patients with pitted keratolysis had hyperhidrosis, and after 10 days of sole treatment with erythromycin 3% topical gel, all 94 patients had a reduction of plantar sweating down to normal limits.[16] These authors hypothesize that hyperhidrosis could be caused by the upregulation of eccrine sweat glands secondary to bacterial infection.[16] Excessive interdigital maceration, secondary to hyperhidrosis, can also develop a bacterial superinfection leading to an erythrasma-like presentation. Malodor and maceration are hallmarks of this condition between the toes. Erythrasma can occur in addition or separate from pitted keratolysis and can easily be examined with a Wood lamp.[17]

There is also an increased risk of viral infections, such as verruca plantaris and verruca vulgaris, and an association with atopic/eczematous dermatitis.[3] The presence of plantar verruca and hyperhidrosis have long been linked. The causative organism responsible for plantar warts, human papilloma virus, thrives in moist environments. In theory, those who suffer from both hyperhidrosis and plantar verruca would benefit from a course of a topical drying agent as part of their overall regimen.

PHARMACOLOGIC TREATMENT OPTIONS

Treatment of plantar hyperhidrosis has used various strategies. The first line of treatment has been application of an antiperspirant, such as topical aluminum chloride.[1] In 2011, Streker and colleagues[1] conducted a study on the effectiveness of two different concentrations of aluminum chloride, 12.5% and 30%, and found that both significantly reduced sweat production in plantar hyperhidrosis in 6 weeks. Because both were effective, they recommend using aluminum chloride 12.5%.[1] Although skin irritation is possible with this treatment, the authors applied the aluminum chloride with a roller and had minimal occurrence of irritant dermatitis, which did not interfere with treatment.[1]

Either as a primary treatment or when aluminum chloride or other antiperspirants have been ineffective or have caused skin irritation, iontophoresis is another treatment option for plantar hyperhidrosis.[18] Iontophoresis allows an ionized substance to pass through intact skin via a direct electrical current. It is used with just tap water, or by adding the anticholinergic, glycopyrrolate.[18] This treatment is appealing because once the patient has the iontophoresis device and is instructed on how to use it, this treatment can be done at home about three times per week.[18] There are three available iontophoresis devices available in the United States: the R.A. Fischer (MD-1a and MD-2; R.A. Fischer, Chatsworth, CA, USA) and the Drionic (Drionic, Ojai, CA, USA).[18] It is not fully understood why iontophoresis is effective for plantar hyperhidrosis, but different theories suggest ion deposition plugging sweat glands, blocking the transmission of sympathetic nerves, or the accumulation of hydrogen ions causing a decrease in pH.[18] There can be mild adverse effects associated with this treatment, such as erythema, vesiculation, burning sensation, pins and needles, and dry skin, but these are managed with moisturizers, petroleum jelly, and reducing the frequency of treatments.[18] This treatment, however, is contraindicated in women who are pregnant, in people who have pacemakers or metal implants, and people with cardiac conditions or epilepsy.[18]

Injectable botulinum toxin A (BTX-A) is another method that has been explored for the treatment of plantar hyperhidrosis, although its use on the plantar surface of feet is still considered off-label use.[11] It is a purified neurotoxin that may be an effective treatment when conservative therapy, such as antiperspirants or iontophoresis, is ineffective.[19] BTX-A is a protein that inhibits presynaptic release of acetylcholine, thereby limiting the sympathetic stimulation of the eccrine sweat glands that causes the excess sweating.[19] Because the eccrine sweat glands are normal in size, number, and density in primary focal hyperhidrosis, botulinum toxin works by inhibiting the overactive postganglionic sympathetic cholinergic fibers innervating them.[11] In a case series by Vlahovic and colleagues,[19] BTX-A has been shown to be an effective treatment of recalcitrant plantar hyperhidrosis, with patients reporting decreased sweating up to 6 months after injection, with a 75% improvement in symptoms. It is recommended that the patient be locally anesthetized with topical lidocaine and an ankle block and/or ice because these injections are painful.[19] Before injecting with the reconstituted BTX-A, Minor iodine starch test (**Figs. 1** and **2**) is done to determine the focal areas of hyperhidrosis, and the noncosmetic version of BTX-A is injected intradermally into spots 2 cm apart in a grid pattern (**Fig. 3**).[19] This treatment is a pregnancy Category C drug and should be avoided in nursing mothers.[11] In a study by Vedoud-Seyedi,[20] of 10 patients (five men, five women), 8 out of 10 patients were satisfied and had a significant decrease in sweating, with the maximum duration of benefits between 3 and 6 months following treatment. In a study by Tamura and colleagues,[15] two patients with both plantar hyperhidrosis and pitted keratolysis were treated with injections of botulinum toxin, and were cured of symptoms within 14 days and were still without symptoms 6 months after treatment.

In addition to topical and injectable pharmacologic treatments, oral glycopyrrolate has been shown to be an effective treatment of hyperhidrosis.[21] Because it is an oral

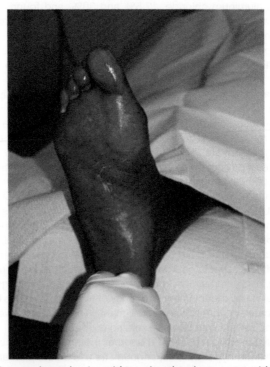

Fig. 1. Minor iodine starch test begins with coating the plantar area with povidone-iodine.

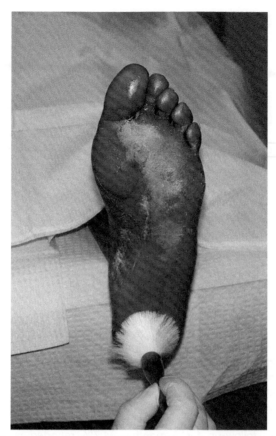

Fig. 2. Minor iodine starch test: after coating the skin with povidone-iodine, corn starch is applied and a color change (povidone-iodine orange to purple) occurs in areas of focal hyperhidrosis.

medication, it works on the whole body and also does not produce any compensatory sweating.[21] Glycopyrrolate is an anticholinergic drug that acts on the nerves innervating sweat glands to decrease sympathetic stimulation and thus decrease sweat production.[21] In a study by Lee and colleagues,[21] in which feet were the second most common area to be affected, 75% of patients had an actual decrease in the amount of sweating, and patients also reported a decrease in discomfort in their everyday lives. Thirty-six percent of patients experienced some side effects, such as oral dryness, palpitations, and headache, but no one stopped taking the medication because of these.[21] This medication is effective in decreasing sweat production without causing too many central side effects because it is a highly polar molecule that does not pass through lipid membranes to the central nervous system.[21] One milligram can be given twice per day, which can be increased up to 8 mg per day.[21]

Oxybutynin is another oral medication that has been explored for the treatment of hyperhidrosis because of its antimuscarinic effects.[22] In a study of children younger than the age of 14 with palmar and plantar hyperhidrosis, 91% reported moderate or great improvement in their level of sweating and almost 95% reported an improvement in their quality of life.[22] Ninety-one percent of these patients reported plantar hyperhidrosis.[22] Patients were given 2.5 mg twice a day for the first

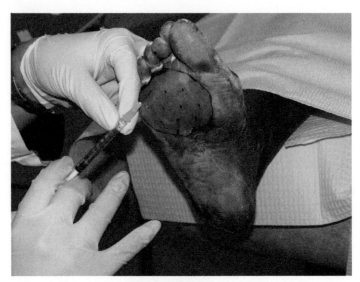

Fig. 3. Injection of BTX-A into the plantar aspect of the foot.

7 days, 2.5 mg twice a day the next 7 days, and then 5 mg twice a day from day 22 to 6 months.[22] The most common side effects was dry mouth, but at 6 weeks, all patients reported moderate or great improvement in sweating levels, and 91% reported the same at 6 months.[22] Of those that had plantar sweating, 90.6% reported moderate or great improvement at 6 months.[22] In another study of the long-term effects of oxybutynin on plantar hyperhidrosis by Wolosker and colleagues,[23] a sample of patients ranging in age from 9 to 71, of the patients that continued to follow-up for 6 months, 84.7% reported moderate or great improvement in self-perceived plantar sweating. The main contraindication for using this medication is glaucoma.[23] Also, patients should be advised that with an oral medication, such as oxybutynin, it can take up to 3 weeks from the start of the medication for the patient to see improvement in symptoms.[23]

NONPHARMACOLOGIC TREATMENT OPTIONS

Laser treatment of hyperhidrosis has been explored for treatment of hyperhidrosis. The miraDry (Miramar Labs, Santa Clara, CA) laser has been tested for treatment of axillary hyperhidrosis, but not plantar hyperhidrosis. It uses microwave energy at 5800 MHz, which is between infrared (CO_2 lasers) and radiowaves on the electromagnetic spectrum.[24] Using an antenna, the microwave energy penetrates the skin to the eccrine sweat glands, preferentially targeting the skin-adipose junction where most eccrine glands are located.[24] The device causes simultaneous cooling because this treatment causes thermolysis of the sweat glands.[24] In a study by Hong and coworkers,[25] this treatment was found to be 90% effective after 12 months with an almost 90% patient satisfaction at 12 months. They found the amount of sweat produced decreased by an average of 82% at 12 months.[25] A total of 90% of patients had at least a 50% reduction in axillary sweat production from baseline.[25] The most common side effects were edema (90%), redness (87%), discomfort (84%), and altered sensation for up to 4 months (45%).[25] The miraDry laser has been shown to be effective in the treatment of axillary hyperhidrosis but again, no studies have been completed for plantar hyperhidrosis at this time.

Aside from nonsurgical treatments, a surgical treatment of plantar hyperhidrosis is endoscopic lumbar sympathectomy.[12] In a study by Rieger and colleagues,[12] 52 patients with primary plantar hyperhidrosis underwent endoscopic lumbar sympathectomy. Of these patients, 96% reported elimination of plantar sweating. Sixty-five percent reported compensatory sweating, which is common after sympathectomies, but 88% reported that they would have the surgery again and 96% were satisfied with their postoperative results, reporting a decrease in plantar sweating and an increase in their quality of life.[12] The International Hyperhidrosis Society does not recommend any type of endoscopic sympathectomy for plantar hyperhidrosis even as a last resort because of the possibility of compensatory sweating in other areas, the irreversible nature of the procedure, heat intolerance, and other potential challenging side effects.[26]

Beyond encouraging patients to wash and dry the feet daily, use drying foot powders, allow shoes to dry out by alternating pairs, and change their socks daily, other nonpharmacologic treatments focus on lifestyle and alternative therapies, which involve everything from shoe gear considerations to holistic therapies, such as hypnosis. The Web site SweatHelp.org has many helpful ideas and Web sites for patients to investigate. Modifying shoe gear, socks, and insoles is a starting point for patients to begin changing their quality of life. Shoe liners that absorb sweat and decrease odor include Summer Soles (Summer Soles, Frisco, TX, USA) and MeshPro Ultra Drying insoles (NanoDri, Japan). Patients should avoid cotton socks that do not wick away moisture and switch to such brands as drymax, Thorlos (Thor-Lon fiber), and Atlas dress socks (Ministry of Supply company, Boston, MA, USA). Many of these insoles and socks listed have research that was performed by the manufacturer. All-leather shoes with no plastic linings and mesh upper soled running sneakers are anecdotally and traditionally recommended by physicians. Alternative therapies, such as hypnosis, biofeedback, and cognitive behavioral methods, have been shown in various cases to be useful for hyperhidrosis across the body, although no specific studies have been used for plantar hyperhidrosis.[27]

SUMMARY/DISCUSSION

Plantar hyperhidrosis has a significant impact on the quality of life for patients. It is important to be able to understand and diagnose this condition, and to be familiar with available treatment options. Determining the cause, if possible, for the hyperhidrosis is paramount before initiating other systemic or more invasive procedures. Evaluating the disruption of the patient's quality of life is useful in determining the treatment plan and understanding the unique needs of the patient with hyperhidrosis. Various treatment methods have been described, but none are specific or all approved for plantar hyperhidrosis. They also offer temporary solutions, unless an underlying condition is the source of the excessive sweating and management of that condition yields a positive response. Considering the patient's quality of life, the clinician should offer ideas for insole, sock, and shoe changes. For the patients who want to manage their condition in a more holistic way in addition to their current medical care, such options as hypnosis, biofeedback, and cognitive behavioral therapy are available.

ACKNOWLEDGMENT

Samantha M. Newstadt, BS for her assistance with this article.

REFERENCES

1. Streker M, Tilmann R, Hagen L, et al. Hyperhidrosis plantaris: a randomized, half-side trial for efficacy and safety of an antiperspirant containing different concentrations of aluminum chloride. J Dtsch Dermatol Ges 2012;10:115–9.
2. Walling HW. Clinical differentiation of primary from secondary hyperhidrosis. J Am Acad Dermatol 2011;64(4):690–5.
3. Walling HW. Primary hyperhidrosis increases the risk of cutaneous infection: a case-control study of 387 patients. J Am Acad Dermatol 2009;61(2):242–6.
4. Lima SO, Aragão JF, Machado Neto J, et al. Research of primary hyperhidrosis in students of medicine of the State of Sergipe, Brazil. An Bras Dermatol 2015;90(5): 661–5.
5. Lear W, Kessler E, Solish N, et al. An epidemiological study of hyperhidrosis. Dermatol Surg 2007;33:S69–75.
6. Ak M, Dincer D, Haciomeroglu B, et al. Temperament and character properties of primary focal hyperhidrosis patients. Health Qual Life Outcomes 2013;11:1–5.
7. Hornberger J, Grimes K, Naumann M, et al. Recognition, diagnosis, and treatment of primary focal hyperhidrosis. J Am Acad Dermatol 2004;51(2):274–86.
8. Kaufmann H, Saadia D, Polin C, et al. Primary hyperhidrosis: evidence for autosomal dominant inheritance. Clin Auton Res 2003;13(2):96–8.
9. Yamashita N, Tamada Y, Kawada M, et al. Analysis of family history of palmoplantar hyperhidrosis in Japan. J Dermatol 2009;36:628–31.
10. Braganca GMG, Lima SO, Neto AFP, et al. Evaluation of anxiety and depression prevalence in patients with primary severe hyperhidrosis. An Bras Dermatol 2014; 89(2):230–5.
11. Weinberg T, Solish N, Murray C. Botulinum neurotoxin treatment of palmar and plantar hyperhidrosis. Dermatol Clin 2014;32(4):505–15.
12. Rieger R, Pedevilla S, Lausecker J. Quality of life after endoscopic lumbar sympathectomy for primary plantar hyperhidrosis. World J Surg 2015;39:905–11.
13. Zheng Y, Yanqing W, Chen H, et al. Analysis of the factors influencing the therapeutic effects of onychomycosis. J Tongji Med Univ 2001;21(3):259–62.
14. Boboschko I, Jockenhöfer S, Sinkgraven R, et al. Hyperhidrose als risikofaktor der tinea pedis. Hautarzt 2005;56(2):151–5.
15. Tamura B, Cucé LC, Souza RL, et al. Plantar hyperhidrosis and pitted keratolysis treated with botulinum toxin injection. Dermatol Surg 2004;30:1510–4.
16. Pranteda G, Carlesimo M, Pranteda G, et al. Pitted keratolysis, erythromycin, and hyperhidrosis. Dermatol Ther 2014;27:101–4.
17. Vlahovic TC, Schleicher SM. Skin disease of the lower extremities: a photographic guide. Malvern (PA): HMP Communications; 2012.
18. Pariser D, Ballard A. Iontophoresis for palmar and plantar hyperhidrosis. Dermatol Clin 2014;32:491–4.
19. Vlahovic TC, Dunn SP, Blau JC, et al. Injectable botulinum toxin as a treatment for plantar hyperhidrosis: a case study. J Am Podiatr Med Assoc 2008;98(2):156–9.
20. Vedoud-Seyedi J. Treatment of plantar hyperhidrosis with botulinum toxin type A. Int J Dermatol 2004;43:969–71.
21. Lee HH, Kim do W, Kim do W, et al. Efficacy of glycopyrrolate in primary hyperhidrosis patients. Korean J Pain 2012;25(1):28–32.
22. Wolosker N, Tievelis MP, Krutman M, et al. Long-term efficacy of oxybutynin for palmar and plantar hyperhidrosis in children younger than 14 years. Pediatr Dermatol 2014;32(5):663–7.

23. Wolosker N, Tievelis MP, Krutman M, et al. Long-term results of the use of oxybu-tynin for the treatment of plantar hyperhidrosis. Int J Dermatol 2015;54:605–11.
24. Jacob C. Treatment of hyperhidrosis with microwave technology. Semin Cutan Med Surg 2013;32:2–8.
25. Chih-Ho Hong H, Lupin M, O'Shaughnessy KF. Clinical evaluation of a microwave device for treating axillary hyperhidrosis. Dermatol Surg 2012;38(5):728–35.
26. Available at: http://www.sweathelp.org/hyperhidrosis-treatments/ets-surgery.html. Accessed March 18, 2016.
27. Shenefelt PD. Biofeedback, cognitive-behavioral methods, and hypnosis in dermatology: is it all in your mind? Dermatol Ther 2003;16:114–22.

Index

Note: Page numbers of article titles are in **boldface** type.

Clin Podiatr Med Surg 33 (2016) 453–465
http://dx.doi.org/10.1016/S0891-8422(16)30045-3
0891-8422/16/$ – see front matter

podiatric.theclinics.com

Printed and bound by CPI Group (UK) Ltd, Croydon, CR0 4YY

03/10/2024

01040392-0016